T0259503

Neutropenia

Editor

CHRISTOPH KLEIN

HEMATOLOGY/ONCOLOGY
CLINICS OF NORTH AMERICA

www.hemonc.theclinics.com

Consulting Editors
GEORGE P. CANELLOS
NANCY BERLINER

February 2013 • Volume 27 • Number 1

ELSEVIER

1600 John F. Kennedy Boulevard • Suite 1800 • Philadelphia, Pennsylvania, 19103-2899

http://www.theclinics.com

HEMATOLOGY/ONCOLOGY CLINICS OF NORTH AMERICA Volume 27, Number 1
February 2013 ISSN 0889-8588, ISBN 13: 978-1-4557-7100-4

Editor: Patrick Manley
Developmental Editor: Donald Mumford

Hematology/Oncology Clinics (ISSN 0889-8588) is published bimonthly by Elsevier Inc., 360 Park Avenue South, New York, NY 10010-1710. Months of issue are February, April, June, August, October, and December. Business and Editorial Offices: 1600 John F. Kennedy Blvd., Ste. 1800, Philadelphia, PA 19103–2899. Customer Service Office: 3251 Riverport Lane, Maryland Heights, MO 63043. Periodicals postage paid at New York, NY and at additional mailing offices. Subscription prices are $367.00 per year (domestic individuals), $599.00 per year (domestic institutions), $179.00 per year (domestic students/residents), $417.00 per year (Canadian individuals), $732.00 per year (Canadian institutions) $496.00 per year (international individuals), $732.00 per year (international institutions), and $241.00 per year (international and Canadian students/residents). International air speed delivery is included in all *Clinics* subscription prices. All prices are subject to change without notice. **POSTMASTER:** Send address changes to *Hematology/Oncology Clinics of North America*, Elsevier Health Sciences Division, Subscription Customer Service, 3251 Riverport Lane, Maryland Heights, MO 63043. Customer Service (orders, claims, online, change of address): Elsevier Health Sciences Division, Subscription Customer Service, 3251 Riverport Lane, Maryland Heights, MO 63043. Tel: 1-800-654-2452 (U.S. and Canada); 314-447-8871 (outside U.S. and Canada). Fax: 314-447-8029. E-mail: journalscustomerservice-usa@elsevier.com (for print support); journalsonlinesupport-usa@elsevier.com (for online support).

Reprints. For copies of 100 or more, of articles in this publication, please contact the Commercial Reprints Department, Elsevier Inc., 360 Park Avenue South, New York, New York 10010-1710; Tel.: 212-633-3813, Fax: 212-462-1935, E-mail: reprints@elsevier.com.

Hematology/Oncology Clinics of North America is covered in *MEDLINE/PubMed (Index Medicus), EMBASE/ Excerpta Medica, and BIOSIS.*

Printed and bound by CPI Group (UK) Ltd, Croydon, CR0 4YY
Transferred to Digital Printing, 2013

Contributors

CONSULTING EDITORS

GEORGE P. CANELLOS, MD
William Rosenberg Professor of Medicine, Department of Medical Oncology, Dana-Farber Cancer Institute, Boston, Massachusetts

NANCY BERLINER, MD
Chief, Division of Hematology, Brigham and Women's Hospital, Professor of Medicine, Harvard Medical School, Boston, Massachusetts

EDITOR

CHRISTOPH KLEIN, MD, PhD
Professor of Pediatrics, Department of Pediatrics, Dr. von Hauner Children's Hospital, University Children's Hospital, Ludwig-Maximilians-University Munich, Munich, Germany

AUTHORS

BLANDINE BEAUPAIN, MSc
Pediatric Hemato Oncology, Hopital Trousseau, Paris, France

RENÉE BEEKMAN, MD
Department of Hematology, Erasmus University Medical Center, Rotterdam, The Netherlands

CHRISTINE BELLANNÉ-CHANTELOT, MD, PhD
Department of Genetics, AP-HP Pitié Salpétriére Hospital, Pierre et Marie Curie University, Paris Cedex, France

KAAN BOZTUG, MD
Department of Pediatrics and Adolescent Medicine, CeMM Research Center for Molecular Medicine of the Austrian Academy of Sciences, Medical University of Vienna, Vienna, Austria

SETH J. COREY, MD, MPH
Department of Pediatrics; Department of Cell and Molecular Biology, Northwestern University Feinberg School of Medicine, Chicago, Illinois

STELLA M. DAVIES, MBBS, PhD, MRCP
Professor of Pediatrics, Division of Bone Marrow Transplantation and Immune Deficiency, Cincinnati Children's Hospital Medical Center, University of Cincinnati, Cincinnati, Ohio

JEAN DONADIEU, MD, PhD
Pediatric Hemato Oncology, Hopital Trousseau, Paris, France

H. LEIGHTON GRIMES, PhD
Division of Immunobiology, Cincinnati Childrens Hospital Medical Center, Cincinnati, Ohio

STEVEN M. HOLLAND, MD
Chief, Laboratory of Clinical Infectious Diseases, National Institute of Allergy and Infectious Diseases, National Institutes of Health, Bethesda, Maryland

MARSHALL S. HORWITZ, MD, PhD
Department of Pathology, University of Washington School of Medicine, Seattle, Washington

CHRISTOPH KLEIN, MD, PhD
Professor of Pediatrics, Department of Pediatrics, Dr. von Hauner Children's Hospital, University Children's Hospital, Ludwig-Maximilians-University Munich, Munich, Germany

TACO W. KUIJPERS, MD, PhD
Emma Children's Hospital, Academic Medical Centre, University of Amsterdam, Amsterdam, The Netherlands

NIZAR MAHLAOUI, MD
Immuno Hematology Unit, Reference Center for Hereditary Immune Deficiency, Necker-Enfants Malades, Assistance Publique-Hôpitaux de Paris, Paris, France

KASIANI C. MYERS, MD
Assistant Professor of Pediatrics, Division of Bone Marrow Transplantation and Immune Deficiency, Cincinnati Children's Hospital Medical Center, University of Cincinnati, Cincinnati, Ohio

KARISHMA PALANDE, PhD
Department of Tumor Immunology, Nijmegen Center for Molecular Life Sciences, Nijmegen, The Netherlands

ALEJANDRO A. SCHÄFFER, PhD
Computational Biology Branch, National Center for Biotechnology Information, National Institutes of Health, Department of Health and Human Services, Bethesda, Maryland

AKIKO SHIMAMURA, MD, PhD
Associate Professor of Pediatrics, Department of Pediatric Hematology/Oncology, Fred Hutchinson Cancer Research Center, Seattle Children's Hospital, University of Washington, Seattle, Washington

JULIA SKOKOWA, MD, PhD
Department of Molecular Hematopoiesis, Children's Hospital, Hannover Medical School, Hannover, Germany

TIMOTHY TIDWELL, BS
Program in Molecular and Cellular Biology, University of Washington School of Medicine, Seattle, Washington

IVO P. TOUW, PhD
Department of Hematology, Erasmus University Medical Center, Rotterdam, The Netherlands

EDITH VAN DE VIJVER, MSc
Emma Children's Hospital, Academic Medical Centre, University of Amsterdam;
Department of Blood Cell Research, Sanquin Research and Landsteiner Laboratory,
Amsterdam, The Netherlands

TIMO K. VAN DEN BERG, PhD
Department of Blood Cell Research, Sanquin Research and Landsteiner Laboratory,
Amsterdam, The Netherlands

KARL WELTE, MD
Department of Molecular Hematopoiesis, Children's Hospital, Hannover Medical School,
Hannover, Germany

Contents

> Epidemiologic investigations of congenital neutropenia aim to determine
> several important indicators related to the disease, such as incidence at
> birth, prevalence, and outcome in the population, including the rate of
> severe infections, leukemia, and survival. Genetic diagnosis is an impor-
> tant criterion for classifying patients and reliably determining the epidemi-
> ologic indicators. Patient registries were developed in the 1990s. The
> prevalence today is probably more than 10 cases per million inhabitants.
> The rate of infection and leukemia risk can now be calculated. Risk factors
> for leukemia seem to depend on both the genetic background and cumu-
> lative dose of granulocyte colony stimulating factor.

> The 2 main forms of hereditary neutropenia are cyclic (CN) and severe con-
> genital (SCN) neutropenia. CN is an autosomal dominant disorder in which
> neutrophil counts fluctuate with 21-day periodicity. SCN consists of static
> neutropenia, with promyelocytic maturation arrest in the bone marrow.
> Unlike CN, SCN displays frequent acquisition of somatic mutations in
> the gene *CSF3R*. CN is caused by heterozygous mutations in the gene
> *ELANE*, encoding neutrophil elastase. SCN is genetically heterogeneous
> but is most frequently associated with *ELANE* mutations. We discuss
> how the mutations provide clues into the pathogenesis of neutropenia
> and describe current hypotheses for its molecular mechanisms.

> Considerable progress has been made in recent years in understanding of
> the genetic basis for congenital neutropenia syndromes. With the advent
> of high-throughput genomic analyzing technologies, the underlying
> genetic causes of other congenital neutropenia syndromes are expected
> to be resolved in the near future. This knowledge will provide the founda-
> tion for genotype-phenotype correlations for infection susceptibility,
> response to therapy, and risk of malignant transformation, enabling opti-
> mal care for individual patients depending on their molecular pathophysi-
> ology. It is hoped that these investigations will enable the development of
> tailored molecular therapies to specifically correct the aberrant signaling
> cascades.

Following activation by their cognate ligands, cytokine receptors undergo intracellular routing toward lysosomes, where they are degraded. This review focuses on the signaling function of the G-CSFR in relation to the dynamics of endosomal routing of the G-CSFR. Mechanisms involving receptor lysine ubiquitination and redox-controlled phosphatase activities are discussed. Specific attention is paid to the consequences of G-CSFR mutations, acquired in patients with severe congenital neutropenias who receive G-CSF therapy, particularly in the context of leukemic transformation, a major clinical complication of the disease.

Several signaling systems downstream of G-CSFR have been identified that are defective or hyperactivated in myeloid cells of patients with congenital neutropenia: severely reduced expression of myeloid-specific transcription factors LEF-1 and C/EBPα, severely reduced expression and functions of HCLS1 protein, severely reduced expression of neutrophil elastase protein, dramatic compensatory up-regulation of the NAMPT/NAD$^+$/SIRT pathway leading to continuous activation of emergency granulopoiesis via the transcription factor C/EBPβ, and hyperactivation of STAT5 protein by tyrosine phosphorylation.

Chronic granulomatous disease (CGD) is a paradigm for nonlymphoid primary immune defects, and has guided elucidation of oxygen metabolism in the phagocyte, vasculature, and brain. It has been in the forefront of the development of antimicrobial prophylaxis before the advent of advanced HIV and before its routine use in neutropenia. It has been an attractive target for gene therapy and bone marrow transplantation for nonmalignant diseases. Therefore, CGD is worthy of attention for its historical interest and because it is a disease for which expert management is imperative.

During inflammation, leukocytes play a key role in maintaining tissue homeostasis through elimination of pathogens and removal of damaged tissue. Leukocytes migrate to the site of inflammation by crawling over and through the blood vessel wall, into the tissue. Leukocyte adhesion deficiencies (ie, LAD-I, -II, and LAD-I/variant, the latter also known as LAD-III) are caused by defects in the adhesion of leukocytes to the vessel wall, resulting in severe recurrent nonpussing infections and neutrophilia, often preceded by delayed separation of the umbilical cord. Although dependent on the genetic defect, hematopoietic stem cell transplantation is often the only curative treatment.

Shwachman–Diamond syndrome (SDS) is an inherited neutropenia syndrome associated with a significant risk of aplastic anemia and malignant transformation. Multiple additional organ systems, including the pancreas, liver, and skeletal and central nervous systems, are affected. Mutations in the Shwachman-Bodian-Diamond syndrome (SBDS) gene are present in most patients. There is growing evidence that SBDS functions in ribosomal biogenesis and other cellular processes. This article summarizes the clinical phenotype of SDS, diagnostic and treatment approaches, and novel advances in our understanding of the molecular pathophysiology of this disease.

In vivo animal models have proven very useful to the understanding of basic biologic pathways of the immune system, a prerequisite for the development of innovate therapies. This article addresses currently available models for defined human monogenetic defects of neutrophil granulocytes, including murine, zebrafish, and larger mammalian species. Strengths and weaknesses of each system are summarized, and clinical investigators may thus be inspired to develop further lines of research to improve diagnosis and therapy by use of the appropriate animal model system.

HEMATOLOGY/ONCOLOGY CLINICS OF NORTH AMERICA

Preface

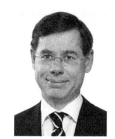

Christoph Klein, MD, PhD
Editor

Neutrophil granulocytes, the most abundant type of white blood cells, have played a major role in medicine and biology, ever since Paul Ehrlich introduced a methodology of staining blood cells prior to microscopic analysis and Ilya Metchnikoff discovered phagocytosis as a prime mechanism of immunity in the late 19th century. For more than 100 years, physicians have been aware that a lack of neutrophil granulocytes predisposes to severe and life-threatening infections. With his landmark discovery of patients with congenital agranulocytis, the pediatrician Rolf Kostmann has laid the groundwork to a field of research that has provided a fascinating spectrum of diseases associated with defective differentiation and/or function of neutrophil granulocytes. Studying rare patients with disorders of neutrophil granulocytes allows us to define basic biological principles governing differentiation and function of a leukocyte subtype that continues to raise questions for clinicians and scientists alike.

This volume provides an overview of our current understanding of rare diseases affecting differentiation, homeostasis, and function of neutrophil granulocytes. The authors address both clinical and basic scientific issues and thus highlight interdisciplinary connections needed to move the field forward. It should not be seen as a completed encyclopedic oeuvre but rather as a work-in-progress report of relevance for physicians and biologists. Clinical and scientific collaborations beyond national and even continental boundaries, often greatly supported by patient groups, have contributed to a great success story that is not yet finished. New nosologic entities continue to be described. Several novel genetic defects have already been discovered and are currently under study. Therapeutic principles are constantly being refined. The authors of this volume share the hope that a better understanding of clinical, epidemiologic,

Hematol Oncol Clin N Am 27 (2013) xi–xii
http://dx.doi.org/10.1016/j.hoc.2012.11.005
0889-8588/13/$ – see front matter © 2013 Published by Elsevier Inc.

hemonc.theclinics.com

cellular, and genetic features will eventually result in the development of better therapies for patients with quantitative and qualitative defects of neutrophil granulocytes.

Christoph Klein, MD, PhD
Department of Pediatrics
Dr von Hauner Children's Hospital
Ludwig Maximilians University Munich
Lindwurmstrasse 4
D-80337 Munich, Germany

E-mail address:
Christoph.Klein@med.uni-muenchen.de

Epidemiology of Congenital Neutropenia

Jean Donadieu, MD, PhD[a],*, Blandine Beaupain, MSc[a],
Nizar Mahlaoui, MD[b], Christine Bellanné-Chantelot, MD, PhD[c]

KEYWORDS

- Congenital neutropenia • Epidemiology • Birth incidence • Prevalence

KEY POINTS

- Congenital neutropenia is a large family of diseases, and genetic diagnosis is an important criterion for classifying patients and reliably determining the epidemiologic indicators.
- Globally, patient registries were developed in the early 1990s to assess the safety of granulocyte colony-stimulating factor (GCSF) and concentrate expertise on the diseases.
- Approximately 20 years after starting the registries, incidence at birth was determined in 2 countries, roughly between 10 and 15 cases per million births, and the prevalence is probably more than 10 cases per million inhabitants.
- The rate leukemia risk can now be calculated reliably. Risk factors for leukemia seem to depend on both the genetic background and cumulative dose of GCSF.

INTRODUCTION

Congenital neutropenia is characterized by chronic neutropenia caused by a constitutional genetic defect. Epidemiologic investigations of congenital neutropenia aim to define the incidence at birth, prevalence, and several complications that occur in the course of the disease, such as lethal infections or leukemia. The management of congenital neutropenia has changed since granulocyte colony-stimulating factor

The French registry is supported by grants from Amgen SAS, Chugai SA, GIS Maladies Rares, Institut de Veille Sanitaire, and Inserm. This project was supported by a grant from Association Laurette Fugain and by constant and unlimited support from the Association Sportive de Saint Quentin Fallavier since 2004, with the unlimited commitment of Mr Gonnot. The authors thank IRIS for its support. This study was conducted by the Center de Reference des Deficits Immunitaires Héréditaires (CEREDIH: the French National Reference Center for Primary Immune Deficiencies, www.ceredih.fr) and was supported by the Société d'Hémato Immunologie Pédiatrique.
[a] Service d'Hémato Oncologie Pédiatrique Registre des neutropénies congénitales, Assistance Publique-Hôpitaux de Paris, Hopital Trousseau 26 Avenue du Dr Netter, Paris F 75012, France; [b] Unité d'Immuno-Hématologie et Rhumatologie pédiatriques, et Centre de référence des déficits Immunitaires Héréditaires (CEREDIH), Groupe Hospitalier Necker-Enfants Malades, Assistance Publique-Hôpitaux de Paris, Paris 75015, France; [c] Département de Génétique, AP-HP Groupe Hospitalier Pitié-Salpêtrière, Université Pierre et Marie Curie, 47/83 Bd de l'Hôpital Bâtiment 10 Lapeyronie, 75651 Paris Cedex 13, France
* Corresponding author.
E-mail address: jean.donadieu@trs.aphp.fr

Hematol Oncol Clin N Am 27 (2013) 1–17
http://dx.doi.org/10.1016/j.hoc.2012.11.003
0889-8588/13/$ – see front matter © 2013 Elsevier Inc. All rights reserved.

(GCSF) became available for commercial use in 1993. Before this date, the literature was composed exclusively of case reports. The largest survey before 1990 involved 16 cases.[1] However, during this period, several entities have been described, including Kostmann disease, Shwachman disease, cyclic neutropenia, glycogen storage disease type Ib, and WHIM syndrome (warts, hypogammaglobulinemia, infections, and myelokathexis syndrome). With its potential risk of leukemia, the availability of GCSF stimulated the development of patient registries. In 1993, such registries were organized in the United States, Canada, France, and Germany, and with the support of Amgen, an International Severe Chronic Neutropenia Registry (ISCNR) encompassing North America and Germany via independent association with public support in France. The establishment of registries allows better definition of diseases and their outcomes. Since the early 1990s, particularly during the last decade, the molecular bases of several entities have been discovered, leading to changes in disease classification. Kostmann syndrome is often considered to be part of the paradigm of congenital neutropenia; it was first described in a Swedish publication in 1950,[2] and subsequently in English in 1956.[3] The syndrome has 3 main characteristics: profound neutropenia (<0.2 G/L) occurring during the first weeks of life, maturation arrest of granulopoiesis at the promyelocyte stage, and death due to bacterial infections. Eleven of the 14 patients in the first report of the disease died in their first year of life from bacterial infections. Nearly 50 years later, a patient's life expectancy routinely exceeds 20 years and the molecular basis of this entity has been identified.[4] Kostmann syndrome is now known to be accompanied by mutation of *HAX1* protein (Kostmann pedigree) and neurologic involvement (mental retardation and epilepsy) if mutation involved 1 of the 2 isoforms of the *HAX1* protein.[5] Thus, the paradigm of congenital neutropenia is early hematologic expression and later neurologic involvement.

Knowledge of the molecular basis of other forms of congenital neutropenia has also modified the disease classification. Until the late 1990s, the literature distinguished between permanent neutropenia (severe congenital neutropenia or Kostmann syndrome) and cyclic neutropenia, which is associated with a regular pattern of change in the neutrophil count, typically every 21 days, with autosomal dominant transmission.[6] This distinction was made based on the International Registry of Chronic Neutropenia,[7,8] in which cyclic neutropenia was not included among the congenital neutropenias. In 1999, Horwitz and colleagues[9] identified mutations in the neutrophil elastase gene (*ELANE*) among 13 pedigrees of patients with cyclic neutropenia. The same team later found that many patients with severe congenital neutropenia also have mutations in *ELANE*.[10] This finding pointed to a continuum between severe congenital neutropenia and cyclic neutropenia, and showed that both can be considered congenital.

The term congenital neutropenia is not used homogeneously in the literature.[11–13] One restrictive definition reserves the term congenital neutropenia for severe forms of the disease that are not associated with immunologic or extrahematopoietic abnormalities, whereas a broader definition includes all diseases that comprise chronic neutropenia, with or without immunologic or extrahematopoietic abnormalities. Thus, only some investigators include glycogen storage disease Ib, Shwachman disease, WHIM syndrome, and Barth disease in the definition of congenital neutropenia.

EPIDEMIOLOGY
Definition of Congenital Neutropenia

Definition of the morbid phenomenon is critical in epidemiology. In this review, the term congenital neutropenia is not restricted to disorders in which neutropenia is the only phenotypic manifestation but encompasses all congenital disorders comprising neutropenia. The authors also consider neutropenia as a continuum, ranging from intermittent forms with various periods of neutrophil deficiency to permanent circulating neutrophil deficiency. **Table 1** provides the list of genetic diseases that we consider congenital neutropenia[14] and for which there is information available in the literature. All of these forms of congenital neutropenia are extremely rare and have monogenic inheritance, which may be X-linked, autosomal, recessive, or dominant. In addition to congenital neutropenia with a documented genetic defect, several patients present with chronic neutropenia of probable genetic origin that is presumably considered congenital neutropenia. This category represents 30% to 50% of patients, depending on the survey, and cannot be considered as marginal. Increased knowledge regarding genetic neutropenia will help to classify the forms of this disease. A category termed idiopathic neutropenia is frequently reported. Patients in this category have chronic neutropenia with no detectable cause. Whether idiopathic neutropenia and congenital neutropenia with no known genetic defect are the same cannot yet be determined, but they are likely the same and the difference just a matter of terminology. In addition to this group of patients, ethnic neutropenia should be considered because it is a congenital neutropenia. Epidemiologic studies have shown that the prevalence of neutropenia (<1.5 g/L) is approximately 4.5% in blacks and 0.8% in whites.[15] Few data are available on other populations, but a high frequency has been noted in the Arabian peninsula,[16] and the frequent mild neutropenia reported in Crete likely corresponds to the same entity.[17] Ethnic neutropenia is not associated with increased susceptibility to infection, and no symptoms have ever been reported. Three simple, but poorly specific, classic features are present: moderate neutropenia (0.5–1.5 g/L), no infection attributable to neutropenia, and no identifiable cause. The few available studies of ethnic neutropenia have yielded strictly normal findings; in particular, the bone marrow is qualitatively and quantitatively normal. A particular polymorphism of the Duffy antigen receptor for cytokines (DARC)[18] is associated with ethnic neutropenia in blacks. Because ethnic neutropenia is not a morbid situation, it is not discussed further, but many ethnic neutropenia cases may be considered idiopathic neutropenia, which causes some misclassification. The ultimate difficulty in defining congenital neutropenia is caused by a genetic defect involving B or T lymphocytes, such as Bruton disease, severe combined immune deficiency (SCID) including peculiar reticular dysgenesis, and several forms of familial hemophagocytic lymphohistiocytosis such as Chediak-Higashi syndrome or Griscelli syndrome type 2. We have excluded these diseases from congenital neutropenia, even though some may actually present neutropenia in the course of the disease or be diagnosed as neutropenia.[14] In addition, we have excluded all types of neutropenia secondary to drugs, viral infection, or autoimmune processes.

What Health Indicators are Useful for Describing Congenital Neutropenia?

Health indicators are not original in congenital neutropenia; they encompass standard indicators such as incidence at birth, prevalence in the overall population, and some well-defined indicators of morbidity, including mortality rate, age at death, and quality of life. More specific to congenital neutropenia is the rate of severe infections, the proportion of patients receiving GCSF, the dose of GCSF used, the number of hematopoietic stem cell transplantations, the rate of severe comorbidity, and the rate of leukemia.

How to Determine Health Indicators and the Role of Registries

Congenital neutropenia is poorly recognized by the public health system. The International Classification of Diseases (ICD) versions 9 and 10 offer some possibilities for coding chronic neutropenia, including codes 284.0, 288.0, 288.2, and 288.5 in ICD9

Table 1
Classification of congenital neutropenia by known genes (2012)

Subgroup of Neutropenia	Disease Name/Reference	OMIM Code	Main Hematologic Features	Other Features	Inheritance	Gene Localization	Gene	Normal Function of the Gene
Congenital neutropenia without extrahematopoietic manifestations	Severe congenital neutropenia/cyclic neutropenia[9,38]	202700 162800	Severe permanent Maturation arrest Intermittent/cyclic with variable bone marrow features	No	Dominant	19q13.3	ELANE	Protease activity Antagonism with α1 antitrypsin
	Severe congenital neutropenia, somatic mutation of CSF3R[66]	202700	Permanent Maturation arrest Unresponsive to GCSF	No	No genetic inheritance	1p35-p34.3	CSF3R	Transmembrane GCSF receptor/intracellular signaling
Congenital neutropenia with innate or adaptive deficiency but no extrahematopoietic features	Severe congenital neutropenia[67]	202700	Permanent/severe or mild Sometimes maturation arrest	Internal ear (in mouse model) Lymphopenia	Dominant	1p22	GFI1	Transcription factor Regulation of oncoprotein
	Severe congenital neutropenia[68,69]	301000	Severe, permanent maturation arrest	Monocytopenia	X-Linked	Xp11.4-p11.21	WAS	Cytoskeleton homeostasis
	WHIM[70]	193670	Severe, permanent No maturation arrest Myelokathexis	Lymphopenia Monocytopenia Warts	Dominant	2q21	CXCR4	Chemokine receptor
	STK4/MTS1[41]		Mild neutropenia, inconstant	Lymphopenia Monocytopenia Warts	Dominant	20q13.12	STK4/ MTS1	Serine/threonine kinase
	GATA2[42,63]	614172 614038	Mild neutropenia No maturation arrest	Monocytopenia Warts	Dominant	3q21.3	GATA2	Transcription factors/zinc finger

Congenital neutropenia with extrahematopoietic manifestations							
Kostmann disease[4,5,71-73]	614038	Maturation arrest	Mental retardation/seizures	Recessive	1q21.3	HAX1	Anti-apoptotic protein located in mitochondria and in the cytosol
Shwachman-Bodian-Diamond disease[34]	601626	Mild neutropenia Dysgranulopoiesis mild dysmegakaryopoeisis	Exocrine pancreatic deficiency Metaphyseal dysplasia Mental retardation Cardiomyopathy	Recessive	7q11.22	SDBS	Ribosomal protein regulation
Severe congenital neutropenia[74]	614286	Maturation arrest	Prominent superficial venous network Atrial defect Uropathy	Recessive	17q21	G6PC3	Glucose-6-phosphatase complex: catalytic unit
Barth disease[75]	302060	No maturation arrest	Hypertrophy Cardiomyopathy	X-Linked	Xq28	TAZ (G4.5)	Tafazzin: phospholipid membrane homeostasis
Hermansky-Pudlak syndrome type 2[76]	608233	No maturation arrest	Albinism	Recessive	5q14.1	AP3B1	Cargo protein/ER trafficking with ELANE interaction
Neutropenia with LAMTOR2 mutation[77]		No maturation arrest	Albinism	Recessive	1q21	LAMTOR2	Lysosome packaging

(continued on next page)

Table 1
(continued)

Subgroup of Neutropenia	Disease Name/Reference	OMIM Code	Main Hematologic Features	Other Features	Inheritance	Gene Localization	Gene	Normal Function of the Gene
	Poikiloderma type Clericuzio[78,79]	604173	No maturation arrest Minor dysgranulopoietic features	Poikiloderma	Recessive	16q13	*16ORF57*	Not known
	Glycogen storage type Ib[80]	232220	No maturation arrest	Hypoglycemia Fasting hyperlactacidemia Glycogen overload of the liver	Recessive	11q23.3	*SLC37A4*	Glucose-6-phosphatase complex: trans ER transporter
	Cohen syndrome[81]	216550	No maturation arrest	Psychomotor retardation Clumsiness Microcephaly Characteristic facial features Hypotonia Joint laxity Progressive retinochoroidal dystrophy Myopia	Recessive	8q22-q23	*VPS13B*	Sorting and transporting proteins in the ER

Abbreviation: ER, endoplasmic reticulum.

and D70 and P61.5 in ICD10, but in practice, large databases, including hospital discharge records and national death records, are not appropriate for identifying patients with congenital neutropenia because congenital neutropenia is not separated from chemotherapy-induced neutropenia, a far more common condition.

Patient registries have been in place for several decades for cancer, birth defects, and cardiovascular diseases, and have been recognized as appropriate tools for improving knowledge about rare diseases[19] in both the European Union (EU)[20] and North America.[21]

Patient registries are the only instruments able to provide epidemiologic knowledge on congenital neutropenia, but a registry is a complex medical organization and its development requires several steps. First, these structures must meet sufficient ethical and administrative criteria according to their national health system. A registry must have technical expertise and computer technology to manage information flow and produce relevant health indicators. Case recruitment and monitoring is also a crucial step, which implies centralization of information and simultaneous contacts with physicians following patients, who are necessarily scattered and not experts in these diseases. The identification of cases is also made difficult by the evolution of the classifications of these diseases, both for the referring physicians and the patients. Thus, development of a registry is a dynamic process that occurs over many years. In each country, these registries have a specific history, usually starting from the commitment of 1 institution and extending to national multisite recruitment. According to the national context, congenital neutropenia can undergo either specific organization or be included in registries built for all types of immunodeficiencies or bone marrow failure. In addition to a large registry aiming to collect all subtypes of congenital neutropenia, some structures are dedicated to a single disease, such as Barth disease[22] or Shwachman-Diamond disease.[23]

The quality of information produced by registries can be classified according to the grading of evidence-based medicine.[24,25] Here, evidence is ranked on 4 levels: A, meta-analyses, high-quality systematic reviews, randomized controlled trials with a low risk of bias; B, systematic reviews of case-control or cohort studies; C, nonanalytical studies, including case reports, case series, and retrospective small studies; D, expert opinion.

ORGANIZATION OF REGISTRIES FOR CONGENITAL NEUTROPENIA

So far, no homogeneous approach exists for a congenital neutropenia registry. In Israel[26] and Canada,[27] patients are included in the registry of bone marrow failure syndrome, but some cases in these countries may be enrolled in the ISCNR.[11] In Sweden and France, a specific structure is dedicated to recording congenital neutropenia cases,[12,28,29] but in France the Severe Chronic Neutropenia Registry also participates in the French National Registry of Primary Immune Deficiency Diseases (CEREDIH)[30] and the European Society for ImmunoDeficiencies (ESID) database.[31] In Iran, congenital neutropenia cases are recorded in a general immunodeficiency registry.[32,33] The ISCNR was funded in 1993 and is dedicated to chronic neutropenia, which includes patients from Australia, North America, and many EU countries, except France. The enrollment by countries remains heterogeneous, with many discrepancies in prevalence by country. According to the standard of evidence-based medicine, the quality of the information produced by registries is still low. Almost all collections of data have to be considered to be grade C with regard to evidence-based medicine criteria, but it is clearly progress from the previous period when no data were collected. A critical issue for all registries is the completeness of cases in a given population.

Incidence at Birth

The incidence at birth is a relevant indicator for a genetic condition. To date, only 2 studies[27,28] have investigated incidence at birth by establishing a ratio between the number of new cases observed during a specified period and the number of births during the same interval. These 2 studies have considered virtually the same diagnostic categories, although the Swedish study considered the diagnostic categories of Pearson syndrome and Griscelli disease among congenital neutropenia. In the Canadian study,[27] a rate of 15.9 cases of congenital neutropenia per million births were reported, whereas the Swedish study[28] reported an incidence rate of 10 cases per million births. The magnitude of these incidence rates seem to be similar at birth, but significant differences emerge for some pathologies, such as Shwachman syndrome, which has an incidence rate of 8.5 cases per million births in Canada and 2.5 cases per million births in Sweden. Thus far, it is difficult to establish if such a difference reflects the genetic background of the studied population rather than some bias interfering in the evaluation.

Prevalence

The prevalence is the number of living patients in a defined geographic area. This indicator is extremely difficult to evaluate because it supposes that all living patients in a given territory can be counted. Another method is to know the exact birth incidence and mean life expectancy for each disease, because it is simply the incidence multiplied by the duration of the disease. It is too early in the development of knowledge about congenital neutropenia to expect reliable information with regard to the prevalence in a population. The evidence does not go above grade B. However, the most recent information from the various patient registries is compared in **Table 2**. Some registries combine congenital neutropenia and idiopathic neutropenia, or even autoimmune neutropenia. Nevertheless, the prevalence rates are heterogeneous and reflect the efficacy of the registry to detect cases in their respective countries. Among the different countries, the highest observed prevalence rate was 9 cases per million inhabitants (France). Such a high rate is probably a minimal value because the coverage of all registries, including the French registry, is less efficient for adult patients, who may have congenital neutropenia. Progress in enrollment into the registry has to occur in all countries to obtain better indicators.

Genetic Epidemiology

Understanding the genetics of congenital neutropenia is not only progress for the pathophysiology of diseases, it is also helpful in classifying patients and allows comparisons between cohorts of patients, offering the possibility of determining the genetic epidemiology of congenital neutropenia. However, 2 minimal conditions are needed to study genetic epidemiology: the gene responsible for a subtype of the diseases has to be known and the patients need to be tested. Such a process takes time to be disseminated worldwide. For a newborn affected by congenital neutropenia, the disease is phenotypically recognized by a doctor, even if the technology is available for diagnosis, then the gene is studied. All of this consideration leads to a delay in detecting cases after birth, in addition to the time needed for the reporting process. This context explains why many patients can remain undiagnosed and why genetic epidemiologic studies of congenital neutropenia are a long process. However, in 2012, it is approximately 10 years since the discovery of 2 important genes relevant to congenital neutropenia: *ELANE* mutations were first reported in 1999[9] and *SBDS* in 2003.[34] These 2 genetic entities are the most frequent in all countries and present in

Table 2
Prevalence of congenital neutropenia and idiopathic neutropenia by country based on registry data

Country	Number of Cases Reported	Congenital Neutropenia (CN) Only or Congenital and Idiopathic	Population in Millions	Estimated Prevalence per Million Inhabitants	Source of Information
Austria	18	CN and idiopathic	8	2.25	EU Registry[a]
Australia	47	CN and idiopathic	22.5	2.1	International Severe Chronic Neutropenia Registry; 2006 report[7,11]
Belarus	3	CN and idiopathic	10	0.3	EU Registry[a]
Belgium	28	CN and idiopathic	10.7	2.6	EU Registry[a]
Canada	60	CN only	33	1.8	Bone Marrow Failure Registry[27]
Croatia	2	CN and idiopathic	4	0.5	EU Registry[a]
Czech Republic	4	CN and idiopathic	10.5	0.3	EU Registry[a]
France	527	CN only	62	8.5	Last report June 2012[12,29]
Germany	224	CN and idiopathic	82	2.7	EU Registry[a]
Greece	12	CN and idiopathic	9.9	1.2	EU Registry[a]
Ireland	12	CN and idiopathic	4.5	2.6	EU Registry[a]
Israel	24	CN only	8	3	Bone Marrow Failure Registry[26]
Italy	44	CN and idiopathic	60.6	0.7	EU Registry[a]
Iran	29	CN and idiopathic	75	0.3	Primary Immunodeficiency Registry[32,33]
Luxembourg	2	CN and idiopathic	0.5	4	EU Registry[a]
Morocco	1	CN and idiopathic	35	0.02	EU Registry[a]
Norway	19	CN and idiopathic	4.9	3.8	EU Registry[a]
Poland	5	CN and idiopathic	38	0.1	EU Registry[a]
Portugal	2	CN and idiopathic	10.7	0.1	EU Registry[a]
Russia	1	CN and idiopathic	143	0.006	EU Registry[a]
Serbia	2	CN and idiopathic	7.3	0.2	EU Registry[a]
Spain	20	CN and idiopathic	47	0.4	EU Registry[a]
Sweden	32	CN only	9.3	3.4	Literature[28]
Switzerland	10	CN and idiopathic	7.8	1.2	EU Registry[a]
Netherlands	14	CN and idiopathic	16.6	0.8	EU Registry[a]
Turkey	19	CN and idiopathic	73	0.2	EU Registry[a]
United Kingdom	66	CN and idiopathic	63	1	EU Registry[a]
United States	685	CN and idiopathic	314	2.1	International Severe Chronic Neutropenia Registry; 2006 report[7,11]

[a] C. Zeidler, communication, June 2012.

roughly 40% of cases. **Table 3** summarizes the patients genotyped for congenital neutropenia in the literature. In the French registry, 20% of the 527 patients had *ELANE* neutropenia (10% severe congenital neutropenia and 10% cyclic neutropenia), 20% had Shwachman-Diamond syndrome, 6% had glycogen storage disease Ib, 4% had Barth disease, 3% had Cohen disease, and 1% to 2% had *HAX1, G6PC3, STK4/MST1,* or *GATA2* mutations, whereas 30% of cases remained undetermined. However, the distribution of the different forms was influenced by the patients' geographic origins (eg, immigrants to Western countries). Some mutations seemed to be linked to geographic origin (*HAX1* in Kurdistan and Sweden, *G6PC3* in Arameans, *LAMTOR2* in Mennonites), whereas *ELANE, SBDS, SLC37A4* (previously named *G6PT1*), and *CXCR4* mutations seem to be spread universally.

OUTCOMES
Risk of Severe Infection

Bacterial infections represent a major risk in congenital neutropenia. Infections can be life threatening or otherwise impair the quality of life, particularly in the case of chronic

Table 3
Congenital neutropenia based on the causative gene and estimated prevalence

Disease Name/ Reference	Gene	Cumulative Number of Cases Reported Worldwide in 2012	References
Severe congenital neutropenia/cyclic neutropenia	*ELANE*	250–500	9,28,38,56,82
Shwachman-Bodian-Diamond disease	*SDBS*	250–500	29,34
Glycogen storage type Ib	*SLC37A4*	150–200	80
Barth disease	*TAZ*	150–200	Barth foundation[22]
Cohen syndrome	*VPS13B*	100–150	81
GATA2	*GATA2*	80–100	42,63
WHIM	*CXCR4*	50–60	39,64,70,83
Severe congenital neutropenia	*G6PC3*	50	74,84
Poikiloderma type Clericuzio	*16ORF57*	50	78,79
Kostmann disease	*HAX1*	40–50	4,5,71–73
Severe congenital neutropenia	*WAS*	40–50	68,69
Severe congenital neutropenia, somatic mutation of CSF3R	*CSF3R*	<5	66
Severe congenital neutropenia	*GFI1*	<5	67
STK4/MTS1	*STK4/MST1*	<5	41
Hermansky-Pudlak syndrome type 2	*AP3B1*	<5	76
Neutropenia with AP14 mutation	*LAMTOR2*	1 family, 4 cases	77

oral infections, leading to recurrent aphthosis, paradontopathy, and tooth loss. The natural risk of life-threatening, invasive infections is high in the absence of any therapy. In the 1950s, almost all patients with the most severe form of the disease, permanent and profound neutropenia, died in the first 2 years of life from sepsis, cellulitis, or pneumonia; this was the case for 11 of the 14 patients in Kostmann's pedigree.[3] Two deaths from pneumonia were reported in a survey of 16 patients with cyclic neutropenia,[35] but no deaths were reported among patients with chronic benign neutropenia.[1,36] In the 1960s and 1970s, lethal sepsis became less frequent with more extensive use of antibiotic therapy, even in the most severe forms of congenital neutropenia. Kostmann's pedigree in 1975 showed long-term survival,[37] and before the GCSF period (since the 1990s), death from infections was already an exception among patients.

In addition to the effect of broad antiinfective therapy, which changed the risk of lethal infections, the risk of infection varies based on several factors. First, the genotype is an important determinant; patients with *ELANE* mutations are exposed to a higher risk of bacterial infections,[38] whereas patients with other subtypes, such as WHIM or Shwachman-Diamond syndrome, have a lower risk.[29,39] Among patients with *ELANE* mutations, the neutrophil count inversely correlates with the risk of sepsis.

Diffuse gastrointestinal lesions are sometimes present, leading to abdominal pain and diarrhea, and sometimes mimicking Crohn disease on radiologic studies.[40] This complication seems to be frequent in glycogen storage disease type Ib.

In addition to the risk of bacterial infections, viral infections or mycobacterial infections may be present, suggesting that neutropenia is associated with a broader immune deficit, such as in WHIM, *STK4/MST1*, *GATA2*,[29,39,41,42] and Shwachman-Diamond disease.[29]

The availability of GCSF since 1988 dramatically changed the medical management of these patients, but lethal bacterial infections are still reported,[12,43] especially in patients with a poor response to GCSF or who have poor compliance. However, chronic stomatologic infection remains difficult to manage, even with GCSF and neutrophil recovery, leading to tooth loss.[44]

Morbidity Related to Extrahematopoietic Involvement

Extrahematopoietic involvement may have a strong impact on patients' lives, including the neurodevelopmental disorders observed in Kostmann disease, Shwachman-Diamond syndrome, and Cohen disease. Cardiac dysfunction may be severe in Shwachman-Diamond syndrome and is almost always observed in Barth syndrome. All these forms of extrahematopoietic involvement increase the burden of chronic disease for both the patient and their family.

Malignant Transformation and Risk Factors

Congenital neutropenias are preleukemic states, which was the major reason for establishing registries at the beginning of the 1990s. Growth factors were first introduced in the late 1980s[45] and have greatly improved the management of chronic neutropenia. After the efficacy of growth factors in neutropenia associated with chemotherapy was demonstrated[46] and the need for long-term administration in some cases emerged,[47] questions about their safety were raised, especially regarding the risk of malignant transformation. The issue was mentioned in the first article reporting the effect of GCSF in this setting,[46] particularly because leukemia had been observed in patients with congenital neutropenia who survived beyond their first decade of life.[48–50]

At that time, the knowledge about congenital neutropenia was limited to phenotype, with large categories, such as Kostmann disease, Shwachman-Diamond disease, cyclic neutropenia, and idiopathic neutropenia. Because GCSF represents an obvious therapeutic improvement for patients, randomization is not possible and registries have simply organized prospective cohorts of patients. The first analysis of these cohorts occurred roughly 10 years after data collection began, and thus far 2 cohorts of patients have provided results: the French registry in 2005[12] and the ISCNR in 2006.[43]

In the French registry at the time of the analysis, 13 cases of leukemia were recorded among 231 patients observed for a total of 3166 person years and in the ISCNR, 44 leukemia cases were recorded among 374 patients observed for a total of 2043 person years. The main difference in the methodologies of the 2 studies was the inclusion of patients who did not receive GCSF in the French registry, whereas all patients in the ISCNR received GCSF.

Despite such differences, a similar conclusion was reached in these 2 studies; GCSF dose is associated with a risk of secondary leukemia. Factors favoring malignant transformation include disease-related factors and GCSF exposure. Disease-related factors comprise the type of neutropenia, because myelodysplasia and leukemia are observed only in patients with severe congenital neutropenia or Shwachman-Diamond syndrome; the severity of neutropenia (ie, the number and severity of infections); the degree of neutropenia; and the level of myeloid arrest in the bone marrow. Two characteristics of GCSF exposure are significantly linked to the risk of leukemic transformation: the cumulative dose and the mean dose per injection. The cumulative duration of GCSF exposure and the length of posttreatment follow-up are not associated with increased risk of leukemia. The relative risk of myelodysplasia and leukemia in patients receiving an average of 15 µg/kg/d GCSF was 5.7 compared with patients who did not receive GCSF. No threshold of exposure below which GCSF does not increase the risk of leukemia has been identified. In addition, the small size of this sample rules out firm conclusions, but patients requiring more than 10 µg/kg per injection and who receive a cumulative dose of more than 10,000 µg/kg clearly have an increased risk of malignant transformation.[12]

The relationship between GCSF exposure and secondary myelodysplasia and leukemia has been obtained in cohort studies of patients with aplastic anemia[51,52] and breast cancer,[53–55] showing that GCSF has a leukemogenic effect in situations that are clearly distinct from congenital neutropenia.

Leukemic transformation is also different with regard to genetic background, such as mutations in ELANE,[12,56] HAX1,[57] WASP,[58] SBDS,[12,59] G6PC3,[60] SLC37A4,[61,62] or GATA2.[42,63] Patients with SBDS and patients with GATA2 mutations have presented with a higher risk of secondary leukemia although they receive less GCSF.

Survival

The survival of patients with congenital neutropenia clearly depends on the care they receive. Overall, the survival rate is approximately 90%, and 80% are now regularly observed in developed countries by 20 years and 30 years of age.[12,28] Older patients are less well documented. Three major causes of early death are observed: sepsis and lethal infections, myelodysplasia and leukemia, and extrahematopoietic failure, such as heart dysfunction in Barth syndrome or Shwachman-Diamond syndrome.

Quality of Life

The impact of the disease on quality of life and professional capacity seems to be important based on clinical experience, but has not been evaluated frequently. Thus far, the quality of life of patients with congenital neutropenia has been evaluated only in 2 ancillary studies of clinical trials of GCSF. The 2 studies involved 10 and 19 patents, who had poor baseline quality of life that improved during GCSF therapy.[64,65]

ACKNOWLEDGMENTS

The authors thank the patients and their families for their participation in this study.

REFERENCES

1. Pincus SH, Boxer LA, Stossel TP. Chronic neutropenia in childhood. Analysis of 16 cases and a review of the literature. Am J Med 1976;61(6):849–61.
2. Kostmann R. Hereditär reticulos - en ny systemsjukdom. Svenska Läkartideningen 1950;47:2861–8.
3. Kostmann R. Infantile genetic agranulocytosis; agranulocytosis infantilis hereditaria. Acta Paediatr Suppl 1956;45(Suppl 105):1–78.
4. Klein C, Grudzien M, Appaswamy G, et al. HAX1 deficiency causes autosomal recessive severe congenital neutropenia (Kostmann disease). Nat Genet 2007; 39(1):86–92.
5. Carlsson G, van't HI, Melin M, et al. Central nervous system involvement in severe congenital neutropenia: neurological and neuropsychological abnormalities associated with specific HAX1 mutations. J Intern Med 2008;264(4):388–400.
6. Palmer SE, Stephens K, Dale DC. Genetics, phenotype, and natural history of autosomal dominant cyclic hematopoiesis. Am J Med Genet 1996;66(4):413–22.
7. Dale DC, Cottle TE, Fier CJ, et al. Severe chronic neutropenia: treatment and follow-up of patients in the Severe Chronic Neutropenia International Registry. Am J Hematol 2003;72(2):82–93.
8. Freedman MH, Bonilla MA, Fier C, et al. Myelodysplasia syndrome and acute myeloid leukemia in patients with congenital neutropenia receiving G-CSF therapy. Blood 2000;96(2):429–36.
9. Horwitz M, Benson KF, Person RE, et al. Mutations in ELA2, encoding neutrophil elastase, define a 21-day biological clock in cyclic haematopoiesis. Nat Genet 1999;23(4):433–6.
10. Dale DC, Person RE, Bolyard AA, et al. Mutations in the gene encoding neutrophil elastase in congenital and cyclic neutropenia. Blood 2000;96(7):2317–22.
11. Dale DC, Bolyard AA, Schwinzer BG, et al. The Severe Chronic Neutropenia International Registry: 10-year follow-up report. Support Cancer Ther 2006;3(4):220–31.
12. Donadieu J, Leblanc T, Bader MB, et al. Analysis of risk factors for myelodysplasias, leukemias and death from infection among patients with congenital neutropenia. Experience of the French Severe Chronic Neutropenia Study Group. Haematologica 2005;90(1):45–53.
13. Notarangelo LD, Fischer A, Geha RS, et al. Primary immunodeficiencies: 2009 update. J Allergy Clin Immunol 2009;124(6):1161–78.
14. Donadieu J, Fenneteau O, Beaupain B, et al. Congenital neutropenia: diagnosis, molecular bases and patient management. Orphanet J Rare Dis 2011;6(1):26.
15. Hsieh MM, Everhart JE, Byrd-Holt DD, et al. Prevalence of neutropenia in the U.S. population: age, sex, smoking status, and ethnic differences. Ann Intern Med 2007;146(7):486–92.
16. Denic S, Showqi S, Klein C, et al. Prevalence, phenotype and inheritance of benign neutropenia in Arabs. BMC Blood Disord 2009;9:3.
17. Papadaki HA, Xylouri I, Coulocheri S, et al. Prevalence of chronic idiopathic neutropenia of adults among an apparently healthy population living on the island of Crete. Ann Hematol 1999;78(7):293–7.
18. Grann VR, Ziv E, Joseph CK, et al. Duffy (Fy), DARC, and neutropenia among women from the United States, Europe and the Caribbean. Br J Haematol 2008;143(2):288–93.

19. Dreyer NA, Garner S. Registries for robust evidence. JAMA 2009;302(7):790–1.
20. Available at: http://nestor.orpha.net/EUCERD/upload/file/RDTFRegistriesrev2011. pdf. Accessed November 29, 2012.
21. Available at: http://rarediseases.info.nih.gov/. Accessed November 29, 2012.
22. Available at: https://www.peds.ufl.edu/barthsyndromeregistry/scientist.htm. Accessed November 29, 2012.
23. Cipolli M, D'Orazio C, Delmarco A, et al. Shwachman's syndrome: pathomorphosis and long-term outcome. J Pediatr Gastroenterol Nutr 1999;29(3):265–72.
24. Atkins D, Eccles M, Flottorp S, et al. Systems for grading the quality of evidence and the strength of recommendations I: critical appraisal of existing approaches The GRADE Working Group. BMC Health Serv Res 2004;4(1):38.
25. Guyatt GH, Oxman AD, Sultan S, et al. GRADE guidelines: 9. Rating up the quality of evidence. J Clin Epidemiol 2011;64(12):1311–6.
26. Tamary H, Nishri D, Yacobovich J, et al. Frequency and natural history of inherited bone marrow failure syndromes: the Israeli Inherited Bone Marrow Failure Registry. Haematologica 2010;95(8):1300–7.
27. Tsangaris E, Klaassen R, Fernandez CV, et al. Genetic analysis of inherited bone marrow failure syndromes from one prospective, comprehensive and population-based cohort and identification of novel mutations. J Med Genet 2011;48(9): 618–28.
28. Carlsson G, Fasth A, Berglof E, et al. Incidence of severe congenital neutropenia in Sweden and risk of evolution to myelodysplastic syndrome/leukaemia. Br J Haematol 2012;158(3):363–9.
29. Donadieu J, Fenneteau O, Beaupain B, et al. Classification and risk factors of hematological complications in a French national cohort of 102 patients with Shwachman-Diamond syndrome. Haematologica 2012;97(9):1312–9.
30. The French national registry of primary immunodeficiency diseases. Clin Immunol 2010;135(2):264–72.
31. Available at: http://www.esid.org/registry-number-of-patients. Accessed November 29, 2012.
32. Rezaei N, Aghamohammadi A, Moin M, et al. Frequency and clinical manifestations of patients with primary immunodeficiency disorders in Iran: update from the Iranian Primary Immunodeficiency Registry. J Clin Immunol 2006;26(6): 519–32.
33. Rezaei N, Moin M, Pourpak Z, et al. The clinical, immunohematological, and molecular study of Iranian patients with severe congenital neutropenia. J Clin Immunol 2007;27(5):525–33.
34. Boocock GR, Morrison JA, Popovic M, et al. Mutations in SBDS are associated with Shwachman-Diamond syndrome. Nat Genet 2003;33(1):97–101.
35. Reimann HA, deBerardinis CT. Periodic (cyclic) neutropenia, an entity; a collection of 16 cases. Blood 1949;4(10):1109–16.
36. Stahlie TD. Chronic benign neutropenia in infancy and early childhood; report of a case with a review of the literature. J Pediatr 1956;48(6):710–21.
37. Kostmann R. Infantile genetic agranulocytosis. Acta Paediatr Scand 1975;64: 362–64368.
38. Bellanne-Chantelot C, Clauin S, Leblanc T, et al. Mutations in the ELA2 gene correlate with more severe expression of neutropenia: a study of 81 patients from the French Neutropenia Register. Blood 2004;103(11):4119–25.
39. Beaussant Cohen S, Fenneteau O, Plouvier E, et al. Description and outcome of a cohort of 8 patients with WHIM syndrome from the French Severe Chronic Neutropenia Registry. Orphanet J Rare Dis 2012;7(1):71.

40. Roe TF, Coates TD, Thomas DW, et al. Brief report: treatment of chronic inflammatory bowel disease in glycogen storage disease type Ib with colony-stimulating factors. N Engl J Med 1992;326(25):1666–9.
41. Abdollahpour H, Appaswamy G, Kotlarz D, et al. The phenotype of human STK4 deficiency. Blood 2012;119(15):3450–7.
42. Hsu AP, Sampaio EP, Khan J, et al. Mutations in GATA2 are associated with the autosomal dominant and sporadic monocytopenia and mycobacterial infection (MonoMAC) syndrome. Blood 2011;118(10):2653–5.
43. Rosenberg PS, Alter BP, Bolyard AA, et al. The incidence of leukemia and mortality from sepsis in patients with severe congenital neutropenia receiving long-term G-CSF therapy. Blood 2006;107(12):4628–35.
44. Carlsson G, Wahlin YB, Johansson A, et al. Periodontal disease in patients from the original Kostmann family with severe congenital neutropenia. J Periodontol 2006;77(4):744–51.
45. Dale DC. The discovery, development and clinical applications of granulocyte colony-stimulating factor. Trans Am Clin Climatol Assoc 1998;109:27–36.
46. Bonilla MA, Gillio AP, Ruggeiro M, et al. Effects of recombinant human granulocyte colony-stimulating factor on neutropenia in patients with congenital agranulocytosis. N Engl J Med 1989;320(24):1574–80.
47. Dale DC, Bonilla MA, Davis MW, et al. A randomized controlled phase III trial of recombinant human granulocyte colony-stimulating factor (filgrastim) for treatment of severe chronic neutropenia. Blood 1993;81(10):2496–502.
48. De Vries A, Peketh L, Joshua H. Leukaemia and agranulocytosis in a member of a family with hereditary leukopenia. Acta Med Orient 1958;17:26–32.
49. Gilman PA, Jackson DP, Guild HG. Congenital agranulocytosis: prolonged survival and terminal acute leukemia. Blood 1970;36:576–85.
50. Rosen R, Kang S. Congenital agranulocytosis terminating in acute myelomonocytic leukemia. J Pediatr 1979;94:406–8.
51. Kojima S, Ohara A, Tsuchida M, et al. Risk factors for evolution of acquired aplastic anemia into myelodysplastic syndrome and acute myeloid leukemia after immunosuppressive therapy in children. Blood 2002;100(3):786–90.
52. Socie G, Mary JY, Schrezenmeier H, et al. Granulocyte-stimulating factor and severe aplastic anemia: a survey by the European Group for Blood and Marrow Transplantation (EBMT). Blood 2007;109(7):2794–6.
53. Hershman D, Neugut AI, Jacobson JS, et al. Acute myeloid leukemia or myelodysplastic syndrome following use of granulocyte colony-stimulating factors during breast cancer adjuvant chemotherapy. J Natl Cancer Inst 2007;99(3):196–205.
54. Le Deley MC, Leblanc T, Shamsaldin A, et al. Risk of secondary leukemia after a solid tumor in childhood according to the dose of epipodophyllotoxins and anthracyclines: a case-control study by the Société Française d'Oncologie Pédiatrique. J Clin Oncol 2003;21(6):1074–81.
55. Smith RE, Bryant J, DeCillis A, et al. Acute myeloid leukemia and myelodysplastic syndrome after doxorubicin-cyclophosphamide adjuvant therapy for operable breast cancer: the National Surgical Adjuvant Breast and Bowel Project Experience. J Clin Oncol 2003;21(7):1195–204.
56. Rosenberg PS, Alter BP, Link DC, et al. Neutrophil elastase mutations and risk of leukaemia in severe congenital neutropenia. Br J Haematol 2008;140(2):210–3.
57. Yetgin S, Olcay L, Koc A, et al. Transformation of severe congenital neutropenia to early acute lymphoblastic leukemia in a patient with HAX1 mutation and without G-CSF administration or receptor mutation. Leukemia 2008;22(9):1797.

58. Beel K, Vandenberghe P. G-CSF receptor (CSF3R) mutations in X-linked neutropenia evolving to acute myeloid leukemia or myelodysplasia. Haematologica 2009;94(10):1449–52.

59. Dror Y. Shwachman-Diamond syndrome. Pediatr Blood Cancer 2005;45(7): 892–901.

60. Stoll C, Alembik Y, Lutz P. A syndrome of facial dysmorphia, birth defects, myelodysplasia and immunodeficiency in three sibs of consanguineous parents. Genet Couns 1994;5(2):161–5.

61. Schroeder T, Hildebrandt B, Mayatepek E, et al. A patient with glycogen storage disease type Ib presenting with acute myeloid leukemia (AML) bearing monosomy 7 and translocation t(3;8)(q26;q24) after 14 years of treatment with granulocyte colony-stimulating factor (G-CSF): a case report. J Med Case Rep 2008;2:319.

62. Pinsk M, Burzynski J, Yhap M, et al. Acute myelogenous leukemia and glycogen storage disease 1b. J Pediatr Hematol Oncol 2002;24(9):756–8.

63. Ostergaard P, Simpson MA, Connell FC, et al. Mutations in GATA2 cause primary lymphedema associated with a predisposition to acute myeloid leukemia (Emberger syndrome). Nat Genet 2011;43(10):929–31.

64. Cleary PD, Morrissey G, Yver A, et al. The effects of rG-CSF on health-related quality of life in children with congenital agranulocytosis. Qual Life Res 1994; 3(5):307–15.

65. Fazio MT, Glaspy JA. The impact of granulocyte colony-stimulating factor on quality of life in patients with severe chronic neutropenia. Oncol Nurs Forum 1991;18(8):1411–4.

66. Ward AC, van Aesch YM, Gits J, et al. Novel point mutation in the extracellular domain of the granulocyte colony-stimulating factor (G-CSF) receptor in a case of severe congenital neutropenia hyporesponsive to G-CSF treatment. J Exp Med 1999;190(4):497–507.

67. Person RE, Li FQ, Duan Z, et al. Mutations in proto-oncogene GFI1 cause human neutropenia and target ELA2. Nat Genet 2003;34(3):308–12.

68. Ancliff PJ, Blundell MP, Cory GO, et al. Two novel activating mutations in the Wiskott-Aldrich syndrome protein result in congenital neutropenia. Blood 2006; 108(7):2182–9.

69. Devriendt K, Kim AS, Mathijs G, et al. Constitutively activating mutation in WASP causes X-linked severe congenital neutropenia. Nat Genet 2001;27(3):313–7.

70. Hernandez PA, Gorlin RJ, Lukens JN, et al. Mutations in the chemokine receptor gene CXCR4 are associated with WHIM syndrome, a combined immunodeficiency disease. Nat Genet 2003;34(1):70–4.

71. Carlsson G, Fasth A. Infantile genetic agranulocytosis, morbus Kostmann: presentation of six cases from the original "Kostmann family" and a review. Acta Paediatr 2001;90(7):757–64.

72. Faiyaz-Ul-Haque M, Al-Jefri A, Al-Dayel F, et al. A novel HAX1 gene mutation in severe congenital neutropenia (SCN) associated with neurological manifestations. Eur J Pediatr 2010;169(6):661–6.

73. Ishikawa N, Okada S, Miki M, et al. Neurodevelopmental abnormalities associated with severe congenital neutropenia due to the R86X mutation in the HAX1 gene. J Med Genet 2008;45(12):802–7.

74. Boztug K, Appaswamy G, Ashikov A, et al. A syndrome with congenital neutropenia and mutations in G6PC3. N Engl J Med 2009;360(1):32–43.

75. Barth PG, Wanders RJ, Vreken P, et al. X-linked cardioskeletal myopathy and neutropenia (Barth syndrome) (MIM 302060). J Inherit Metab Dis 1999;22(4): 555–67.

76. Huizing M, Scher CD, Strovel E, et al. Nonsense mutations in ADTB3A cause complete deficiency of the beta3A subunit of adaptor complex-3 and severe Hermansky-Pudlak syndrome type 2. Pediatr Res 2002;51(2):150–8.
77. Bohn G, Allroth A, Brandes G, et al. A novel human primary immunodeficiency syndrome caused by deficiency of the endosomal adaptor protein p14. Nat Med 2007;13(1):38–45.
78. Mostefai R, Morice-Picard F, Boralevi F, et al. Poikiloderma with neutropenia, Clericuzio type, in a family from Morocco. Am J Med Genet A 2008;146A(21):2762–9.
79. Volpi L, Roversi G, Colombo EA, et al. Targeted next-generation sequencing appoints c16orf57 as Clericuzio-type poikiloderma with neutropenia gene. Am J Hum Genet 2010;86(1):72–6.
80. Veiga-da-Cunha M, Gerin I, Chen YT, et al. The putative glucose 6-phosphate translocase gene is mutated in essentially all cases of glycogen storage disease type I non-a. Eur J Hum Genet 1999;7(6):717–23.
81. Kolehmainen J, Black GC, Saarinen A, et al. Cohen syndrome is caused by mutations in a novel gene, COH1, encoding a transmembrane protein with a presumed role in vesicle-mediated sorting and intracellular protein transport. Am J Hum Genet 2003;72(6):1359–69.
82. Xia J, Bolyard AA, Rodger E, et al. Prevalence of mutations in ELANE, GFI1, HAX1, SBDS, WAS and G6PC3 in patients with severe congenital neutropenia. Br J Haematol 2009;147(4):535–42.
83. Tassone L, Notarangelo LD, Bonomi V, et al. Clinical and genetic diagnosis of warts, hypogammaglobulinemia, infections, and myelokathexis syndrome in 10 patients. J Allergy Clin Immunol 2009;123(5):1170–3, 1173.e1–3.
84. Boztug K, Rosenberg PS, Dorda M, et al. Extended spectrum of human glucose-6-phosphatase catalytic subunit 3 deficiency: novel genotypes and phenotypic variability in severe congenital neutropenia. J Pediatr 2012;160(4):679–83.

ELANE Mutations in Cyclic and Severe Congenital Neutropenia
Genetics and Pathophysiology

Marshall S. Horwitz, MD, PhD[a],*, Seth J. Corey, MD, MPH[b,c],
H. Leighton Grimes, PhD[d], Timothy Tidwell, BS[e]

KEYWORDS

- Cyclic neutropenia • Severe congenital neutropenia • *ELANE* • Neutrophil elastase
- Granulocyte-colony stimulating factor (G-CSF)

KEY POINTS

- Heterozygous mutations in the gene *ELANE*, encoding neutrophil elastase, cause cyclic neutropenia and are the most common cause of severe congenital neutropenia.
- Although many mutations are known, they all result in a translated polypeptide, indicating that it is not merely haploinsufficiency of the enzyme that is responsible for neutropenia.
- Two competing but not mutually exclusive hypotheses suggest that protein mislocalization or protein misfolding may contribute to the pathophysiology of neutropenia.

INTRODUCTION

Normal neutrophil counts in peripheral blood typically range between 1500 to 8500 cells/μL after the age of 1 year,[1] although they vary among individuals from different parts of the world and at different ages. "Benign ethnic neutropenia" has been used to describe the normally lower neutrophil levels observed in certain populations, including African Americans and some Middle Eastern groups.[2] Within individuals, neutrophil counts fluctuate in response to environmental and host factors[3] and to circadian cycles.[4]

[a] Department of Pathology, University of Washington School of Medicine, 850 Republican Street, Seattle, WA 98109, USA; [b] Department of Pediatrics, Northwestern University Feinberg School of Medicine, 303 East Superior Street, Chicago, IL 60611, USA; [c] Department of Cell and Molecular Biology, Northwestern University Feinberg School of Medicine, 303 East Superior Street, Chicago, IL 60611, USA; [d] Division of Immunobiology, Cincinnati Children's Hospital Medical Center, 3333 Burnet Avenue, Cincinnati, OH 45229, USA; [e] Program in Molecular and Cellular Biology, University of Washington School of Medicine, 850 Republican Street, Seattle, WA 98109, USA
* Corresponding author.
E-mail address: horwitz@uw.edu

Hematol Oncol Clin N Am 27 (2013) 19–41
http://dx.doi.org/10.1016/j.hoc.2012.10.004

HERITABILITY OF NEUTROPHIL COUNTS

Total white blood cell counts, which are largely reflective of the number of neutrophils, are moderately heritable.[5] The Duffy Antigen Receptor for Chemokine (*DARC*) gene is at least partly responsible for the lower neutrophil counts observed in individuals of African ancestry[6–8] and is associated with resistance to malaria.[7] Several recent genome-wide association studies (GWAS)[9–11] confirmed association of neutrophil counts in people of African descent with single nucleotide polymorphisms in linkage disequilibrium with *DARC* on chromosome 1q and identified a locus on chromosome 17q among individuals of European descent, in addition to other genetic regions. (It may be coincidental, but it is interesting that *HAX1* and *G6PC3*, whose mutations cause SCN, as described later, are located in proximity to the regions identified in GWAS on chromosomes 1q [nearby *DARC*] and 17q, respectively. However, the area of chromosome 19p where *ELANE* is located has not emerged in GWAS of neutrophil counts.)

MENDELIAN FORMS OF NEUTROPENIA

In contrast to the genetically influenced benign variation in neutrophil numbers arising in the general population are distinct, "Mendelian" neutropenic disorders exhibit highly penetrant single gene autosomal dominant, autosomal recessive, or X-linked inheritance.

Historically, there have been 2 primary classes of hereditary neutropenia. The first is cyclic neutropenia (sometimes referred to as cyclic hematopoiesis), in which neutrophil counts oscillate with approximately 21-day periodicity, fluctuating between nearly normal levels and a nadir lasting several days that often reaches zero.[12] Early descriptions of cyclic neutropenia date to the first half of the twentieth century.[13,14] The periodicity of the neutrophil cycling is exemplified by an unusual case[15] in which a child with acute lymphoblastic leukemia received an allogeneic bone marrow transplant from her sister, who, along with other members of the family, was afflicted with cyclic neutropenia. The recipient was cured of leukemia but developed cyclic neutropenia, which she had not inherited at birth. Remarkably, the neutrophil counts for the 2 sisters subsequently cycled synchronously on the same days of the calendar. Monocytes also cycle in these patients, but their counts typically do so in a phase that is opposite that of neutrophils. Because monocyte counts are typically much lower than neutrophils counts, the cycling is also less apparent, probably because of greater variation in sampling errors with serial blood counts. Nearly all cases of cyclic neutropenia are autosomal dominant or represent de novo autosomal dominant mutations in *ELANE*, which encodes neutrophil elastase.[16]

Description of the second major type of hereditary neutropenia is generally attributed to Kostmann, who in 1956 described a now eponymous syndrome of noncyclical "infantile agranulocytosis" observed among families residing in a remote area of northern Sweden.[17–19] Individuals with this disorder demonstrate noncyclical severe neutropenia with a characteristic arrest of granulocytic differentiation at the promyelocyte stage evident on bone marrow examination.[20] Although a substantial portion of the disorder now most often referred to as SCN is the result of allelic, heterozygous (and therefore dominantly acting) mutations in *ELANE* (which sometimes overlap the mutations observed in cyclic neutropenia),[16] it is now known that SCN represents a genetically heterogeneous group of disorders.[21] The mutated genes include those encoding the HAX1, G6PC3, WAS, GFI1, STK4, and tafazzin proteins (**Table 1**).

Although indistinguishable in their degree of neutropenia compared with SCN caused by *ELANE* mutations, the various autosomal recessive or X-linked forms of

Table 1
Genetic Causes of Human Neutropenia

Disease	Affected Gene	Manner of Inheritance	Syndromic
Cyclic neutropenia	*ELANE*	AD	No
Severe chronic neutropenia	*ELANE*	AD	No
Severe chronic neutropenia	*CSF3R*	AD	No
Severe chronic neutropenia	*HAX1*	AR	Yes, neurodevelopmental features
Severe chronic neutropenia	*G6PC3*	AR	Yes, congenital heart disease and other features
Severe chronic neutropenia	*GFI1*	AR	Yes, lymphocyte abnormalities
Severe chronic neutropenia	*STK4*	AR	Yes, lymphopenia, congenital heart disease
Neutropenia	*SBDS*	AR	Yes, Shwachman-Diamond syndrome
Neutropenia	*RMRP*	AR	Yes, cartilage-hair hypoplasia syndrome
Neutropenia	*SLC37A4*	AR	Yes, glycogen storage disease 1b
Severe chronic neutropenia	*WAS*	X-linked	No (different from Wiskott Aldrich syndrome)
Severe chronic neutropenia	*TAZ*	X-linked	Yes, Barth syndrome

SCN display nonhematologic clinical features depending on the responsible gene.[22] For example, *HAX1*-associated SCN is frequently accompanied by neurodevelopmental complications, including decreased cognitive function and seizures.[23] Individuals with *G6PC3* mutations frequently have congenital heart disease and other clinical features.[24] Patients with mutations in *GFI1* display a range of alterations in lymphocyte numbers or function.[25,26] In contrast, patients with either SCN or cyclic neutropenia resulting from *ELANE* mutations lack associated syndromic features not immediately relatable to disturbance of neutrophil numbers or function, presumably because expression of *ELANE*, in contrast to the case for *HAX1* or *G6PC3* and other genes, is mainly restricted to myeloid progenitor cells.[27] Recently, though, neutrophil elastase was found to be expressed in smooth muscle cells derived from neointimal lesions in mice and humans with pulmonary vascular disease.[28]

An important clinical feature of SCN that largely differentiates it from cyclic neutropenia is the risk for disease progression to myelodysplasia (MDS) and/or acute myeloid leukemia (AML).[29–31] In one series, the cumulative incidence of MDS/AML was 31%,[31] and although leukemia is anecdotally observed with cyclic neutropenia,[32] its occurrence is uncommon. Leukemic transformation arising with hereditary bone marrow failure syndromes is well described and not unique to SCN; it is found at similar frequency, for example, in Shwachman-Diamond syndrome.[33] However, a unique feature of leukemic progression in SCN is the strong (although not completely invariant) association with acquired mutations of the gene *CSF3R*, encoding the granulocyte-colony stimulating factor (G-CSF) receptor.[34] (Although typically encountered as somatic mutations, there is at least one case report of SCN arising from germline *CSF3R* mutation.[35]) Although this is the subject of another article in this issue by Ivo Touw, there are concerns that treatment with recombinant human G-CSF (rhG-CSF) elevates risk for malignant transformation in SCN,[29] particularly in light of the strong association with somatic mutations of the G-CSF Receptor gene and the demonstration in mice that SCN-associated G-CSFR mutations confer clonal dominance only with administration of exogenous G-CSF.[36]

FUNCTIONAL DEFICIENCY OF NEUTROPHILS IN ADDITION TO NEUTROPENIA

An often overlooked property of cyclic neutropenia and SCN is that there are likely functional deficiencies of the neutrophils that may contribute to the risk for infection even in addition to the neutropenia observed in such individuals. Electron microscopy of myeloid progenitor cells from patients with SCN reveals ultrastructural abnormalities in the formation of neutrophil primary granules containing the hydrolytic enzymes responsible for effecting antimicrobial defense.[37] Neutrophils from patients with SCN are deficient in antimicrobial peptides, including α-defensins.[38] Reduced abundance of transcripts encoding other neutrophil granule components is also reported.[39,40] A largely successful form of treatment of cyclic neutropenia and SCN involves administration of rhG-CSF, which increases neutrophil counts in most subjects to within the normal range. However, neutrophils recovered from the peripheral blood from treated patients with SCN display abnormalities in the maturation of granules, and the neutrophils are functionally deficient in antimicrobial activity against fungal and bacterial pathogens.[41] This may be reflected in the types of organisms that are encountered by individuals with cyclic neutropenia and SCN, who may exhibit vulnerability to uncommon pathogens.[42,43] On the other hand, the phenomenon is not necessarily a unique feature of SCN. When neutrophils are collected from CD34+ cells from peripheral blood from healthy donors then expanded ex vivo in the presence of a cytokine cocktail including G-CSF, the resulting neutrophils similarly exhibit reduced quantities of granule components, including neutrophil elastase, and limited bactericidal activity.[44]

Osteoporosis[45] and other bone mineralization defects[46,47] are seen in SCN, although they may be a side effect of treatment with rhG-CSF.[48,49] G-CSF administration reduces bone mineral density by activating osteoclasts[50] and inhibiting osteoblasts.[51] Bone remodeling could conceivably also be secondary to effects of dysregulated neutrophil production and/or activation in the bone marrow microenvironment.

DISCOVERY OF MUTATIONS IN ELANE IN CYCLIC NEUTROPENIA AND SEVERE CONGENITAL NEUTROPENIA

In the late 1990s, our group in Seattle performed genome-wide analysis for genetic linkage in 13 families with multiple generations of individuals affected with cyclic neutropenia, using the then-current technology of microsatellite markers, distributed with mean separation of approximately 10-cM genetic distance.[52] In every family, we observed genetic linkage to markers mapping near the distal terminus of the short arm of chromosome 19, where obvious candidate genes included a cluster of 3 paralogous serine chymotryptic-type proteases, ELANE (then known as ELA2) encoding neutrophil elastase; PRTN3 encoding proteinase 3, which is the target of "c-ANCA" (cytoplasmic antineutrophil cytoplasmic antibodies) autoantibodies associated with the rheumatologic disorder Wegener's granulomatosis; and NAZC encoding azurocidin, in which the catalytic serine has disappeared, resulting in a protein that no longer displays proteolytic activity. It is worth noting that these proteins display antimicrobial activity distinct from their enzymatic activity.[53] After sequencing this cluster of genes, we detected 7 different heterozygous mutations in ELANE that segregated with cyclic neutropenia in each of the 13 families we studied.[52]

We next evaluated ELANE as a candidate gene in 27 SCN unrelated cases.[54] In 21 of the 27 cases, we detected 1 of 15 different heterozygous ELANE mutations. Many of the cases occurred sporadically, but when DNA samples from other affected individuals in the family were available, in nearly all cases when there was evidence of parent-to-child transmission, consistent with autosomal dominant forms of inheritance, the same *ELANE* mutation was detected in all members of a pedigree. For the most part, *ELANE* mutations occurring in patients with SCN are distinct from those found in patients with cyclic neutropenia. Nevertheless, at times the same particular mutation is found in individuals with decidedly clinically distinct forms of neutropenia (ie, cyclic versus chronic). There are several possible explanations. First, the clinical evaluation of cyclic neutropenia can be challenging, because observing cycles requires frequent serial blood counts. Oscillation patterns may exhibit irregularity, may disappear entirely at times, and are influenced by therapy, particularly rhG-CSF treatment, which tends to shorten the periodicity of cycling and increase the amplitude of the cycles, without abrogating cycling completely. Some individuals may cycle but exhibit low peak amplitudes resulting in a classification of SCN. Another possibility is that the clinical assignment was made in light of knowledge of the mutation, so genotype-phenotype correlations could conceivably be biased as a result of knowledge of the particular mutation. Finally, there is some recent evidence to suggest that there could be modifier genes and that the modifiers might themselves include variants of *ELANE*, *HAX1*, and *G6PC3*.[55] In particular, 2 individuals with SCN who seemed to be heterozygous for a pathogenic mutation in *ELANE* were also heterozygous for either *HAX1* or *G6PC3* mutations. (Ordinarily, *HAX1* and *G6PC3* act recessively, and homozygous mutation is thought to be required to produce the SCN phenotype.) Another patient was a compound heterozygote for 2 different pathogenic *HAX1* mutations but was also heterozygous for a *G6PC3* mutation. Finally, one other SCN patient was heterozygous for both *G6PC3* and *HAX1* mutations. It is worth emphasizing that although recessive forms of SCN are rare, consideration of Hardy-Weinberg equilibrium indicates that carriers are markedly more common, raising the possibility that heterozygosity for *HAX1* or *G6PC3* is an incidental finding in these cases. In another study,[56] 2 patients with SCN had novel variants in *GFI1*, which can also be a cause of SCN (see later). In yet another study, an SCN patient was found to have 2 *ELANE* amino acid missense substitution mutations (V53M and V69M), both occurring in *cis* on the maternally inherited allele.[57] The mother, however, exhibited only one of the variants (V69M, which has not apparently been seen before in either cases or controls) and was asymptomatic with normal neutrophil counts. (There was also a third variant within an intron whose parental inheritance, if any, was uncertain.) Thus, V53M must have arisen de novo. It is interesting that V53M had only previously been found in patients with cyclic neutropenia.[16,58] The authors therefore concluded that the combination of V69M, which alone had no effect on granulopoiesis (as found in the mother), with the V53M mutation, ordinarily producing cyclic neutropenia, yielded SCN with a particularly severe clinical course, including invasive pulmonary mycosis and development of MDS with progression to AML at age 8 years.

Another suggestion of modifier genes comes from an unusual case in which a healthy sperm donor fathered (at least) 8 neutropenic children with 6 different women.[59,60] Seven of the 8 children had SCN, whereas one of the children demonstrated evidence of neutrophil cycling. The authors interpreted this observation as indicating phenotype determination by modifying genes, given that all the affected children inherited the same paternal allele. (Sanger dideoxy DNA sequence analysis of the father's sperm was consistent with mosaic representation of the *ELANE* mutation. See further discussion of genetic mosaicism later.)

As noted, de novo mutation of *ELANE* is fairly common,[16] more so among SCN than among cyclic neutropenia cases. In fact, the occurrence of de novo *ELANE* mutation complicated the search for autosomal recessive forms of SCN. There are individuals with SCN residing in Sweden who are descendants of the cases first reported by

Kostmann more than 50 years ago. The gene responsible for autosomal recessive SCN in this population, *HAX1*, was mapped by linkage analysis and positionally cloned by making use of this Swedish family as well as other families from ethnically isolated populations in the Middle East.[61] Four members of Kostmann's original family with SCN were studied. Although 3 were found to be homozygous for the same *HAX1* mutation, one individual whose disease was thought to be clinically indistinguishable from that of his affected siblings (and therefore was attributed to the same ancestral gene) evidently lacked the segregating *HAX1* mutation and was reported to have a new *ELANE* mutation not present in his parents.[62] This is not a genetically surprising phenomenon, given that disorders with reduced reproductive fitness—noting that severe infectious complications, as well as the risk for leukemic progression, severely shorten life—must necessarily arise from new mutations, because affected individuals are less likely to survive to reproductive age. Nevertheless, it is possible that *ELANE* may represent a hotspot or new germline mutation. We have reported several cases in which there have been 2 de novo substitutions occurring in *cis* on the same allele of *ELANE*, representing a phenomenon that has only been extremely rarely reported for other disorders.[63] In the 2 cases we described in which the origin of the mutation could be determined, the mutations had arisen on paternally inherited alleles. This could possibly reflect vulnerability of this locus to mutational phenomenon or, by analogy to study of de novo *FGFR3* mutations causing achondroplasia and other new mutations showing paternal bias, it could reflect selective advantage during male germ cell formation.[64] Arguing against that possibility, though, is the previously discussed case of another patient with 2 *cis ELANE* mutations[57]; one was de novo and one was inherited, but both came from the mother.

The phenomenon of de novo mutation leads to discussion of the significance of germline mosaic *ELANE* mutations. It is now well recognized that in a variety of autosomal dominant disorders, unaffected individuals lacking evidence of the mutation in DNA obtained from peripheral blood or epithelial or other cells obtained via buccal swab or skin biopsy may be a parent to multiple children exhibiting the disorder and sharing a common mutation (the aforementioned sperm donor being one such example). In such cases, the "transmitting" parent is understood to harbor the mutation in only a fraction of the cells required to exhibit symptoms in the relevant tissue (eg, bone marrow for neutropenic disorders) yet sufficiently populates the germline so that its inheritance follows Mendelian expectations.[65]

In fact, documentation of such "germline mosaicism" has allowed for drawing some interesting conclusions about how *ELANE* mutations cause neutropenia. In the first instance in which germline mosaicism was reported,[66] an unaffected father was found in peripheral blood from his DNA to demonstrate the same *ELANE* mutation as present in his affected child. Closer inspection revealed that the mutation was detectable in about half of his lymphocytes but less than 10% of neutrophils. Individual hematopoietic colonies obtained from peripheral blood were either heterozygous for the mutation or homozygous wild-type. One suggested explanation for this and other demonstrated or likely cases of *ELANE* mosaicism[59,67,68] was that it must mean that *ELANE* mutations are, by themselves, not causative of neutropenia.[67] We think, however, that a more probable—and provocative—conclusion is just the opposite: that neutrophil progenitors bearing the mutation do not eventuate in mature neutrophils yet are unable to block differentiation of wild-type cells.[69,70] These observations implicate cell autonomous phenomenon instead of involvement of paracrine effects, at least with respect to how mutations in *ELANE* lead to SCN, if not also to cyclic neutropenia.

ELANE GENE MUTATIONS

It is, first, worth noting that the pathogenic role of *ELANE* mutations in hereditary forms of neutropenia has been repeatedly called into question.[21,60,68] We find this baffling. Families with cyclic neutropenia or SCN exhibit clear-cut multigenerational patterns of inheritance consistent with single gene autosomal dominant transmission. The initial linkage analysis identified just a single locus in 13 of 13 pedigrees with cyclic neutropenia, and *ELANE* mutations, some different and some recurrent yet appearing on different ancestral haplotypes (meaning that they arose independently within the population), were detected in all 13 families.[52] Since then, hundreds of patients with either cyclic neutropenia or SCN who have *ELANE* mutations have been identified[58,71,72]—to list but just a few of the many cases reported in the literature. Multiple examples of de novo mutation of *ELANE*, which is generally accepted as evidence of causality—particularly when examining only a single gene, are now known. Cases of germline mosaicism are also consistent with a causative role. Commercial genetic testing has become routine. Finally, as whole genome or whole exome sequencing becomes increasingly common and databases of common variants are compiled by sequencing thousands of controls,[73] other causative genes can be excluded and the absence of the observed *ELANE* mutations from control populations can be confirmed. We assert that there are few other genes for which the evidence of causality is so strong.

THE NATURE OF THE MUTATIONS OBSERVED IN *ELANE* ALSO PROVIDES CLUES ABOUT THEIR PATHOGENICITY

ELANE contains 5 exons. All known *ELANE* chain-terminating mutations (nonsense or frameshift mutations leading to altered reading frames with incorrect translation of an out-of-frame stop codon) occur in the fifth and final exon. (Chain-terminating mutations within *ELANE* are, for the most part, confined to patients with SCN and are not observed with cyclic neutropenia.) Although chain-terminating mutations occurring within internal exons generally produce transcripts that are selectively removed before translation through the process of nonsense-mediated decay and therefore do not produce an abbreviated polypeptide, mutations occurring in the final exon are typically exempted from such cellular quality control mechanisms and do actually lead to peptides truncated at the carboxyl terminus.[74] This important observation leads to 2 significant conclusions. First, haploinsufficiency of neutrophil elastase is unlikely to be causative of the disorder; otherwise, chain-terminating mutations or whole gene deletions, which have never been observed, should be expected in the first 4 exons. Second, the carboxyl-terminal portion of the polypeptide likely contributes functionally to prevent neutropenia (as discussed later, potentially a binding site for adapter protein 3 (AP3), involved in intracellular trafficking of neutrophil elastase).

Initially, shortly after the discovery of *ELANE* mutations in cyclic neutropenia and SCN, there seemed to be possible clustering patterns related to either the lineal or tertiary distribution of mutations with respect to gene and protein structure, respectively, that predicted their occurrence within either subtype of inherited neutropenia. Potential correlation between mutation location and phenotype has substantially weakened[75] as the number of unique mutations has grown as genetic analysis of *ELANE* has become increasingly common in the evaluation of early childhood neutropenia. Mutations, typically single base missense substitutions or small in-frame indels or splice site mutations producing in-frame deletion or insertion of a few amino acid residues, are now found distributed throughout the length of the gene, rendering any clear pattern, if one actually exists, less obvious (**Fig. 1**). It has become difficult to maintain an accurate database of the various mutations now described because

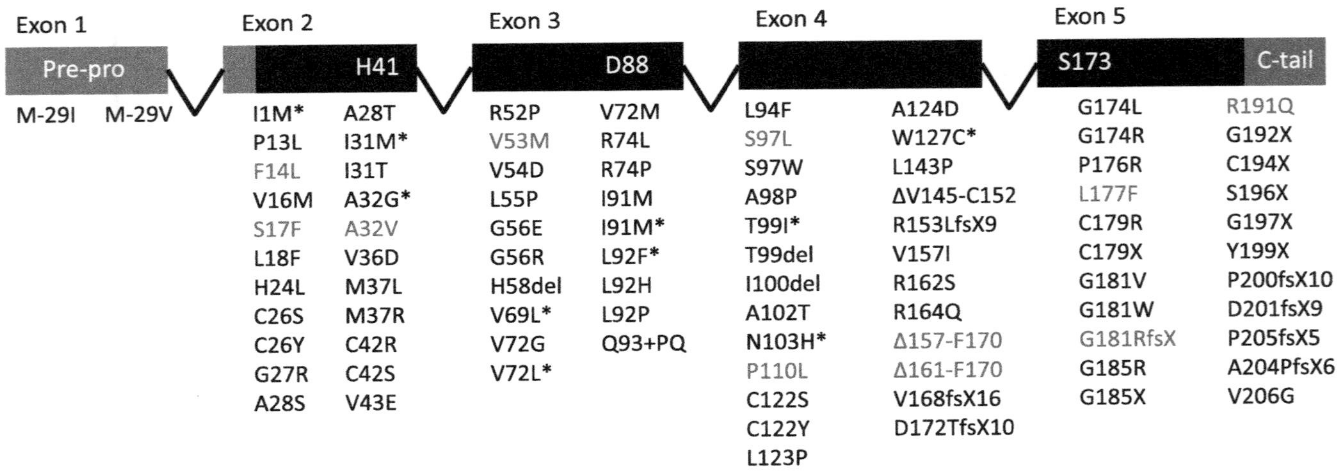

Exon 1 — Pre-pro

- M-29I
- M-29V

Exon 2 — H41

- I1M*
- P13L
- F14L
- V16M
- S17F
- L18F
- H24L
- C26S
- C26Y
- G27R
- A28S
- A28T
- I31M*
- I31T
- A32G*
- A32V
- V36D
- M37L
- M37R
- C42R
- C42S
- V43E

Exon 3 — D88

- R52P
- V53M
- V54D
- L55P
- G56E
- G56R
- H58del
- V69L*
- V72G
- V72L*
- V72M
- R74L
- R74P
- I91M
- I91M*
- L92F*
- L92H
- L92P
- Q93+PQ

Exon 4

- L94F
- S97L
- S97W
- A98P
- T99I*
- T99del
- I100del
- A102T
- N103H*
- P110L
- C122S
- C122Y
- L123P
- A124D
- W127C*
- L143P
- ΔV145-C152
- R153LfsX9
- V157I
- R162S
- R164Q
- Δ157-F170
- Δ161-F170
- V168fsX16
- D172TfsX10

Exon 5 — S173, C-tail

- G174L
- G174R
- P176R
- L177F
- C179R
- C179X
- G181V
- G181W
- G181RfsX
- G185R
- G185X
- R191Q
- G192X
- C194X
- S196X
- G197X
- Y199X
- P200fsX10
- D201fsX9
- P205fsX5
- A204PfsX6
- V206G

Fig. 1. Schematic of mutations of *ELANE* associated with SCN and cyclic neutropenia. Amino acids listed in white represent the catalytic triad active site. Mutations in red are primarily associated with cyclic neutropenia but some have also been reported in SCN. Asterisks denote mutations that are seen in conjunction with a second mutation, always *cis* when determinable.

of the plurality of research and commercial laboratories performing testing. Still, some general observations regarding the nature of the mutations hold. The splice donor site at intron 4 is perhaps the most frequent site at which mutations occur.[16] Base substitutions at the first, third, or fifth position of the intron force use of a cryptic splice donor site 30 nucleotides upstream of the canonical site, leading to deletion of 10 amino acid residues from within a region of the protein containing the catalytic site (Δ161-F170). These mutations are nearly exclusively found in individuals with cyclic neutropenia and are the overwhelmingly most common mutations, with respect to their common effect on protein coding, in cases of cyclic neutropenia. In addition to the observation of chain-terminating mutations in the final exon being nearly exclusively found among patients with SCN, a fairly commonly seen mutation, G815R, seems to confer a particularly severe clinical course.[58,76] Individuals with this mutation tend to have lower neutrophil counts, are refractory to rhG-CSF treatment, and seem to progress to MDS and/or AML at high frequency.

BIOCHEMISTRY OF NEUTROPHIL ELASTASE

ELANE encodes neutrophil elastase, a monomeric approximately 30-kDa glycoprotein.[53] As noted, neutrophil elastase is closely related to azurocidin and proteinase 3, which are encoded by adjacent genes in the same cluster on chromosome 19p. All 3 enzymes are also closely related to cathepsin G, whose gene is found on a different chromosome (14q). All 4 proteins are major component of neutrophil azurophilic granules.

Neutrophil elastase takes its name from the fact that the connective tissue protein elastin was among the first of its known substrates[77]; however, neutrophil elastase claims a large number of different proteins among its substrates. Its ability to accept virulence factors from a variety of Gram-negative bacterial species[78] as substrates, including the outer membrane protein of *E coli*,[79] contributes to its antimicrobial activity.

Neutrophil elastase is also involved in the processing of cytokines, chemokines, and growth factors, including tumor necrosis factor-α[80] and stromal cell–derived factor-1α (also referred to as CXCL12),[81] which serves as a chemoattractant for lymphocytes, monocytes, and dendritic cells. It is interesting that inactivation of patients with stromal cell–derived factor-1α in mice leads to deficient myelopoiesis,[82] and inactivation of its receptor, CXCR4, is the cause of the WHIM syndrome (warts, hypogammaglobulinemia, infections, and myelokathexis).[83] In the WHIM syndrome, peripheral neutropenia is a consequence of myelokathexis, the retention of neutrophils within the bone marrow. Of unknown relevance to SCN, neutrophil elastase also cleaves G-CSF and its receptor.[84–86]

Neutrophil elastase is synthesized as a 267-amino-acid residue inactive zymogen. It is posttranslationally processed to first remove a 27-residue "pre" signal sequence required for intracellular membrane insertion and ultimately extracellular secretion.[87] Then a "pro" peptide of just 2 amino acids is removed from the amino terminus by dipeptidyl peptidase I (also known as cathepsin C).[88] Neutrophil elastase also contains a carboxyl-terminal propeptide of 20 residues that is cleaved by an as-yet-unidentified protease. Fully processed mature neutrophil elastase contains 218 amino acid residues. Unlike other serine proteases, such as trypsin, in which proteolytic conversion from zymogen to active enzyme yields 2 intertwined polypeptides, the processed portions of neutrophil elastase are not found to associate with the resulting mature single protein chain.[89] Regarding posttranslational modifications, neutrophil elastase contains 2 sites of *N*-glycosylation.[53]

Deficiency of DPPI, responsible for cleaving the 2-residue propeptide of neutrophil elastase, causes an autosomal recessive human disorder, Papillon-Lefevre syndrome, consisting of skin and periodontal disease.[90] Individuals with Papillon-Lefevre syndrome therefore fail to appropriately excise the carboxyl-terminal propeptide domain from neutrophil elastase, proteinase 3, cathepsin G, and azurocidin but yet are not described as neutropenic.

Neutrophil elastase's tertiary structure is composed of 2 β-barrels, containing 6 anti-parallel β-sheets connected through a linker segment, and a carboxyl-terminal α-helical domain.[91] As with other serine proteases, there is a triad of catalytic residues (S195, D102, and H57) forming a "charge relay" system.[53] Initially, the histidine is deprotonated by the carboxylate side chain of aspartate. The histidine, in turn, deprotonates serine. The proton originally bound to the serine hydroxyl group is transferred to the amino group in the substrate's peptide bond, allowing the histidine to accept a proton from water, which then attacks the acyl enzyme intermediate, leading to reformation of the enzyme.

Neutrophil elastase and related chymotryptic serine proteases have several endogenous inhibitors. Most prominent perhaps are the serpins (serine proteinase inhibitors), of which the most well-characterized is α1-protease inhibitor (also known as α1–anti-trypsin, but which may play a more significant role in inhibiting neutrophil elastase). Human genetic deficiency of α1-protease inhibitor leads to early onset of emphysematous lung disease, resulting from unopposed neutrophil elastase–mediated destruction of pulmonary elastic fibers and other connective tissues.[92] Certain genetic variants of α1-protease inhibitor can also cause cirrhosis because of their ability to misfold and form protein aggregates that prove toxic to hepatocytes.[93] Among other serpins, monocyte neutrophil elastase (now referred to as SerpinB1) seems to account for a substantial portion of physiologic inhibition of neutrophil elastase.[94] Serpins achieve inhibition of neutrophil elastase and other serine proteases through an irreversible suicide substrate mechanism in which the targeted enzyme cleaves the serpin and generates a covalently bound inhibitory complex.[95] "Canonical inhibitors," including elafin[96] and secretory leukocyte protease inhibitor,[97] form another group of endogenous inhibitors of neutrophil elastase and related serine proteases. Although encoded by different gene families, they share a canonical formation of their inhibitory protease binding loop.

FAILURE OF MOUSE GENETIC MODELS TO RECAPITULATE NEUTROPENIA

A factor hampering the understanding of the mechanism whereby human mutations result in neutropenia is the lack of correspondence to human phenotypes in mouse genetic models. Gene targeting of human *ELANE* mutations at orthologous positions in murine *Elane* fail to produce aberrant granulopoiesis.[98] Similarly, mice genetically deficient in *Hax1* are also not neutropenic, but instead exhibit lymphocytopenia and neuronal cell death.[99] There seem then to be species-specific differences in granulopoiesis. However, not all mouse models are failures in this regard. The impetus for screening *GFI1* as a candidate gene for human SCN (see later) came from observations of neutropenia in *Gfi1* knockout mice.[100,101] The introduction of human SCN patient-associated mutations into murine *Gfi1* coding sequences and forced expression in murine bone marrow progenitors block granulopoiesis,[102] providing the first biologic proof in an animal model for a human neutropenia-associated mutation. Finally, although *G6PC3* was identified as an SCN gene using a genome-wide linkage strategy,[24] *G6pc3*-deficient mice had previously been found to be neutropenic.[103]

HYPOTHESES FOR PATHOGENICITY: GENERAL CONSIDERATIONS

The distinctive neutrophil count oscillations in cyclic neutropenia have attracted considerable attention. Theoretical models of varying levels of mathematical complexity have been proposed.[104,105] A common element to some models involves disturbance of a feedback loop.[106] Abnormal responses to G-CSF or accelerated cell loss through apoptosis affecting the hematopoietic stem cell may be one example of an autoregulatory loop.[107] A feedback model we favor[16] supposes that mature neutrophils elaborate an inhibitor of myelopoiesis whose concentration depends on the numbers of neutrophils present. In normal operation, if peripheral destruction of neutrophils in response to infection, inflammation, or other stress leads to their consumption, then low levels of the inhibitor will allow myelopoiesis to proceed. Once levels of neutrophils have adequately risen, the inhibitor would presumably dampen further production. If there were a perturbation in this circuit such that the hypothesized mediator (or the pathways on which it acted) had its "gain" set at too high a level, then neutrophil production would be overly inhibited—but only for a while because the inhibitor's synthesis is itself dependent on neutrophil production. One can imagine how this would lead to a cyclical pattern.

In fact, there is support for such a "chalone" model, as it was once termed,[108,109] that precedes the discovery of the role of mutations in neutrophil elastase in hereditary forms of neutropenia. A search for molecules possessing predicted inhibitory capacity leads to purification of a neutrophil membrane fraction.[110] The active component within the fraction could be suppressed with chemical inhibitors of neutrophil elastase, yielding the hypothesis that neutrophil elastase was itself the chalone responsible for governing steady state levels of neutrophils.[85] Although it is attractive to hypothesize that a defective chalone could yield an overly sensitive feedback circuit, a potential problem lies in the observation of an absence of neutropenia among individuals who are genetically mosaic for neutrophil elastase mutations (as discussed earlier). In this special circumstance, the presence of the mutation in some myeloid precursors is insufficient to impair production of neutrophils from progenitor cells lacking the mutation. Although the observation seems to rule out the possibility that neutrophil elastase could be acting as a diffusible factor, it does not exclude the potential for it having a more local, if not completely cell autonomous effect, within the bone marrow microenvironment. Nevertheless, because details of such a model necessarily remain conjectural, it is best, in our opinion, to work toward pathophysiologic explanation of inherited neutropenia by building on observations about the consequences of the mutations.

LACK OF BIOCHEMICAL CONSISTENCY

The mutations have varied effects on measurable biochemical activities of neutrophil elastase. Although most reduce or abrogate biochemical activity, a few of the reported mutations lead to apparently fully functional enzyme.[111] Among mutations retaining proteolytic activity, there is no measurable difference in sensitivity to α1-protease inhibitor.[111] There is similarly lack of consistency as to whether mutations affect glycosylation.[112] Theoretical modeling of the mutations has also not identified likely perturbations common to known mutations.[75] No simple hypothesis based on consistent biochemical properties is therefore evident as a likely explanation for how the mutations lead to disease.

MISLOCALIZATION HYPOTHESIS

In addition to being localized within neutrophil granules, neutrophil elastase is secreted and is found on the cell surface,[113–116] as well as being detected within the nucleus.[26,117–122] Although we at one time proposed that neutrophil elastase might be an integral transmembrane protein,[123] in light of other evidence, it seems more likely that neutrophil elastase attaches to the plasma membrane via electrostatic interactions,[53] in particular, with sulfate-containing proteoglycans.[124] We initially proposed that mislocalization of mutant neutrophil elastase might contribute to disease pathogenesis based on several observations. Foremost among them was the molecular genetic elucidation of a similar disease in dogs, canine cyclic neutropenia.[125,126]

Despite their seeming similarities, there are phenotypic differences between human and canine cyclic neutropenia. The human disorder is autosomal dominant, but the canine disease is autosomal recessive. The cycle length in dogs is between 10 and 12 days, instead of the 21-day periodicity observed in humans. The canine disorder is largely confined to the collie breed, where it also results in characteristic coat color dilution, giving rise to its common name, "gray collie syndrome." Most important, the disorders occur because of mutations in 2 different genes in the 2 different species. ELANE is intact in collies; instead, homozygous mutations are found in AP3B1 encoding the β subunit of the adapter protein 3 complex.[123] In humans, mutation of AP3B1 produces Hermansky-Pudlak syndrome type 2.[127]

Hermansky-Pudlak syndromes are genetically heterogeneous disorders typically consisting of partial albinism and platelet granule deficiencies leading to a bleeding diathesis. Among at least 9 known types of human disease (and an even larger number of murine types of this disorder), only type 2 is associated with neutropenia. Although there are not many known human cases, none of those have been described as having cyclical neutropenia; instead. their neutrophil counts seem to be chronically low. Another distinguishing feature in comparison to human SCN arising from ELANE mutations is that no patients with Hermansky-Pudlak syndrome type 2 (or dogs with canine cyclic neutropenia) have been reported as developing MDS or AML.

Despite the fact that canine cyclic neutropenia actually proved to be an animal model for a different human disease, it may nevertheless offer some insight into the pathogenesis of human cyclic neutropenia. AP3 is involved in the trafficking of cargo proteins from the trans-Golgi network to lysosomes,[128] which, in neutrophils, consist of granules. Among its well-characterized cargo proteins is tyrosine hydroxylase, which fails to appropriately localize within melanosomes. The affected melanosomes may be thought of as a sort of specialized lysosomal compartment within melanocytes and account for the pigmentary phenotype in Hermansky-Pudlak syndrome type 2.[129]

We entertained the hypothesis that neutrophil elastase could serve as an AP3 cargo protein. This hypothesis is supported because, in AP3-deficient dogs with canine cyclic neutropenia, neutrophil elastase's distribution is altered as measured by immunofluorescent localization patterns within the cell and by biochemical fractionation.[123,130] Further, neutrophil elastase in neutrophils from dogs affected with canine cyclic neutropenia is not fully proteolytically processed.[130] A yeast 2-hybrid system used for testing potential AP3 cargo protein interactions reveals a potential association between neutrophil elastase and AP3.[9] Importantly, the region of neutrophil elastase responsible for this interaction is within the processed carboxyl terminus, which is recurrently deleted in chain-terminating SCN mutations. Moreover, analysis in cultured cells[9] and neutrophils obtained from patients with ELANE mutations[112] reveals that mutant neutrophil elastase is mislocalized within the cell, again as evidenced by immunofluorescent staining patterns and biochemical fractionation.

Corollary support for this hypothesis comes from similar observations in Chédiak-Higashi syndrome. Humans with Chédiak-Higashi syndrome also have partial albinism and commonly have neutropenia.[131] It is caused by mutations in the LYST gene, which encodes a protein regulating lysosomal trafficking.[132] Corresponding mutation of Lyst in mice is responsible for the beige strain. Beige mice are deficient in neutrophil chemotaxis and bactericidal activity; although they are not neutropenic, significantly, neutrophil elastase is aberrantly subcellularly localized in beige mice.[133,134] (As far as we aware, there has been no study examining whether neutrophil elastase is aberrantly localized in human Chédiak-Higashi syndrome.) It thus seems that mislocalization of neutrophil elastase either via mutation of neutrophil elastase itself or in proteins regulating its lysosomal transport can produce neutropenia, at least in humans. (Oddly enough, Chédiak-Higashi syndrome has been described in at least 6 species,[135] and, although mice with Chédiak-Higashi syndrome are not neutropenic, at least one other species—cats—in addition to humans, is neutropenic.[136] These observations support the view that there are species-specific differences in granulopoiesis that allow for different neutropenic phenotypes in the presence of identical genetic defects.)

Another gene responsible for SCN, albeit rarely, but offering potential support for the mislocalization hypothesis, is *GFI1*, encoding a transcription factor involved in maintenance of hematopoietic stem cells.[137] As noted previously, gene-targeted mice deficient in *Gfi1* were initially reported as having neutropenia.[100,101] More precisely, in addition to lymphopenia and other lymphocyte abnormalities, the mice failed to produce mature neutrophils and monocytes in the peripheral blood but instead showed scant numbers of cells demonstrating an intermediary phenotype. Screening *GFI1* as a candidate gene in otherwise unexplained cases of SCN has led to the identification of occasional mutations in this gene.[25,26,56] The human phenotype closely resembles the mouse phenotype in that the peripheral neutrophils exhibit an immature morphology, as well as lymphocyte abnormalities consistent with those observed in mice. Myeloid progenitor cells exhibit deficiencies in the appearance of granulocytes in colony formation assays. Intriguingly, although *GFI1* targets many genes for transcriptional regulation, both repression and activation, *ELANE* is a target of its transcriptional repression,[25,138] and there are elevated levels of *ELANE* and its translated product, neutrophil elastase, in people and mice deficient in *Gfi1*. One possibility is simply that overexpression of neutrophil elastase overwhelms normal intracellular trafficking pathways and leads to its accumulation in cellular compartments where it is not ordinarily found (or overwhelms endoplasmic reticulum [ER] folding pathways, as described later).

(One case involving germline mutation of *GFI1* is quite remarkable.[5] A young man developed cyclic neutropenia as an adult and was found to have 2 *cis* de novo *GFI1* mutations [both of the mutations described in different patients in another report[25]]. Neutrophil elastase seemed mislocalized from the granules to the nucleus of his neutrophils. Moreover, he showed T-lymphocyte immunity to proteinase 3 and neutrophil elastase, and autoimmune destruction of his neutrophils was thought to be the cause of his cylic neutropenia.)

The mislocalization hypothesis, however, suffers from the finding that not all neutrophil elastase mutations have demonstrable effects on the protein's subcellular localization; moreover, there are not necessarily clean divisions between the alternate destinations of the enzyme (ER retention, accumulation at or near the cell surface, excessive granular deposition, and possibly nuclear presence) and the phenotype (cyclic neutropenia versus SCN) associated with particular mutations.

UNFOLDED PROTEIN HYPOTHESIS

An alternative hypothesis for the pathogenic effects of the various neutrophil elastase mutations takes inspiration from how mutations in one of its inhibitors, α1-protease inhibitor, produces hepatotoxicity.[93] Link and colleagues[72] and Kollner and colleagues[112] have posited that the mutations cause the nascent polypeptide to misfold, thereby inducing a stress response, largely coordinated within the ER, which leads to apoptosis. Indeed, there is substantial support for this hypothesis in cell models of the disorder in which particular mutations are expressed in cultured cells and found to induce markers of ER stress response, including expression of immunoglobulin heavy chain-binding protein (BiP)/78,000-dalton glucose-regulated protein (GRP78) and splicing of X-box-binding protein 1 (XBP1) mRNA.[139] Additional support for this hypothesis derives from study of transgenic mice carrying a targeted mutation of *Elane* (G193X) found in human SCN, which produces a truncated polypeptide.[140] As with other mouse models, the mice initially failed to yield a neutropenic phenotype. However, treatment with the proteasome inhibitor bortezomib, which among other effects results in inhibition of ER-associated degradation pathways, did evoke a neutropenic phenotype. A supportive observation from human genetics involves Wolcott-Rallison syndrome. That disorder is caused by mutations in *EIF2AK3*, a kinase for translation initiation factor-2, which functions as a proximal sensor of ER stress. Disruption of *EIF2AK3* produces ER stress in pancreatic β-islet cells, thereby eventuating in early-onset diabetes mellitus.[141] It is notable that many patients with Wolcott-Rallison syndrome exhibit neutropenia.[142] When mice containing the G193X allele of *Elane* were crossed with *Eif2ak3*-deficient mice, there was, however, no neutropenia or other apparent effects on granulopoiesis. Although this may not be entirely surprising in light of the failure of most mouse genetic models to recapitulate a neutropenic phenotype corresponding to the equivalent human disorder, it does raise the possibility that nonspecific effects of bortezomib's chemical inhibition of the proteasome[143] might be contributing to neutropenia in these experiments. An additional concern is that, as with the other hypotheses advanced to explain how *ELANE* mutations eventuate in neutropenia, not all mutations are capable of consistently experimentally evoking the unfolded protein response. The unfolded protein response hypothesis has additionally yet to offer insight into distinguishing between how different *ELANE* mutations might produce either cyclic neutropenia or SCN, based on the properties of the mutant protein. Finally, it should be emphasized that the mislocalization hypothesis and the unfolded protein hypothesis are not mutually exclusive. Indeed, in the earliest report of induction of the unfolded protein response by Kollner and colleagues,[112] it was thought that aberrant cytoplasmic localization was associated with, if not required, for induction of the stress response.

   Another challenge to the unfolded protein hypothesis is to explain why it is that only mutations in neutrophil elastase are found in human neutropenia. Conceivably, mutations of the closely related proteinase 3 or azurocidin, whose genes lie adjacent to *ELANE* and are similarly prominent granule components, have not been detected. However, to date, no mutations of these genes have been reported.

CHALLENGES POSED BY TRANSLATION INITIATION MUTATIONS

Workers at our laboratory and others[58] have found patients with SCN who have mutations in the initiator methionine codon at the first translated residue encoded by *ELANE*. At first glance, such mutations are problematic in light of other hypotheses. These alleles should not produce a polypeptide and therefore contradict observations based on an absence of gene deletion mutations suggesting that haploinsufficiency of neutrophil elastase causes neutropenia. Moreover, they are incompatible with both the mislocalization and the misfolding hypotheses. (If there is no mutant protein to be made, then how can it mislocalize or misfold?) Our preliminary studies indicate that these mutations force translation from downstream internal initiation codons, which would otherwise encode internal methionine residues, and produce a polypeptide truncated at the amino terminus. We find that some of these internally translated polypeptides are also intracellularly mislocalized. (Our preliminary studies show it accumulating in the nucleus.) It is more difficult to imagine how these peptides could invoke the ER stress response, because their effect is to delete the signal sequence required for targeting to the ER. Further study of this unusual class of mutations is likely to be informative.

CELLULAR CONSEQUENCES OF THE MUTATIONS

Whatever the biochemical consequence of mutant neutrophil elastase, it must somehow translate into a failure of neutrophil maturation. Only a few explanations for neutropenia are tenable: neutrophil progenitors can stop proliferating, they can die, or they can differentiate into an alternate fate. The last possibility is intriguing in light of the reciprocal relationship between neutrophil and monocyte counts in both cyclic neutropenia and SCN. With respect to cell death, intriguingly, some of the earliest electron microscopy studies of cyclic neutropenia demonstrated aberrant promyelocyte granule formation accompanied by autophagy,[144] and several of the genes causing SCN can induce cell death.[21]

Multiple outstanding questions remain: What accounts for how mutations in the same gene, *ELANE*, can produce 2 different forms of neutropenia (cyclic versus SCN) and why, for that matter, is cycling present at all? Importantly, how does pharmacologic administration of rhG-CSF improve granulocyte counts? Another important question that is far from being answered is why do MDS and AML develop in SCN but usually not in cyclic neutropenia? A recent report of multistep evolution of AML from SCN with an *ELANE* mutation during a 17-year period involved the acquisition of 5 distinct *CSF3R* mutations, with 3 of them disappearing.[71] Compared with other leukemia-predisposing bone marrow failure syndromes, why are mutations in the gene encoding the G-CSF receptor such a common feature in SCN? And, does pharmacologic administration of rhG-CSF promote clonal outgrowth of the mutated receptor? No doubt that answers to such questions, should and when they come, will be broadly relevant to both normal and malignant hematopoiesis.

REFERENCES

1. Manroe BL, Weinberg AG, Rosenfeld CR, et al. The neonatal blood count in health and disease. I. Reference values for neutrophilic cells. J Pediatr 1979; 95(1):89–98.
2. Haddy TB, Rana SR, Castro O. Benign ethnic neutropenia: what is a normal absolute neutrophil count? J Lab Clin Med 1999;133(1):15–22.
3. Nieto FJ, Szklo M, Folsom AR, et al. Leukocyte count correlates in middle-aged adults: the Atherosclerosis Risk in Communities (ARIC) study. Am J Epidemiol 1992;136(5):525–37.
4. Sennels HP, Jorgensen HL, Hansen AL, et al. Diurnal variation of hematology parameters in healthy young males: the Bispebjerg study of diurnal variations. Scand J Clin Lab Invest 2011;71(7):532–41.
5. Pilia G, Chen WM, Scuteri A, et al. Heritability of cardiovascular and personality traits in 6,148 Sardinians. PLoS Genet 2006;2(8):e132.
6. Grann VR, Ziv E, Joseph CK, et al. Duffy (Fy), DARC, and neutropenia among women from the United States, Europe and the Caribbean. Br J Haematol 2008;143(2):288–93.
7. Reich D, Nalls MA, Kao WH, et al. Reduced neutrophil count in people of African descent is due to a regulatory variant in the Duffy antigen receptor for chemokines gene. PLoS Genet 2009;5(1):e1000360.

8. Grann VR, Bowman N, Joseph C, et al. Neutropenia in 6 ethnic groups from the Caribbean and the U.S. Cancer 2008;113(4):854–60.

9. Nalls MA, Couper DJ, Tanaka T, et al. Multiple loci are associated with white blood cell phenotypes. PLoS Genet 2011;7(6):e1002113.

10. Reiner AP, Lettre G, Nalls MA, et al. Genome-wide association study of white blood cell count in 16,388 African Americans: the Continental Origins and Genetic Epidemiology Network (COGENT). PLoS Genet 2011;7(6):e1002108.

11. Crosslin DR, McDavid A, Weston N, et al. Genetic variants associated with the white blood cell count in 13,923 subjects in the eMERGE Network. Hum Genet 2012;131(4):639–52.

12. Lange RD. Cyclic hematopoiesis: human cyclic neutropenia. Exp Hematol 1983; 11(6):435–51.

13. Reimann HA. Periodic disease; a probable syndrome including periodic fever, benign paroxysmal peritonitis, cyclic neutropenia and intermittent arthralgia. J Am Med Assoc 1948;136(4):239–44.

14. Borne S. Cyclic neutropenia in an infant. Pediatrics 1949;4(1):70–8.

15. Krance RA, Spruce WE, Forman SJ, et al. Human cyclic neutropenia transferred by allogeneic bone marrow grafting. Blood 1982;60(6):1263–6.

16. Horwitz MS, Duan Z, Korkmaz B, et al. Neutrophil elastase in cyclic and severe congenital neutropenia. Blood 2007;109(5):1817–24.

17. Kostmann R. Infantile genetic agranulocytosis; agranulocytosis infantilis hereditaria. Acta Paediatr Suppl 1956;45(Suppl 105):1–78.

18. Kostmann R. Infantile genetic agranulocytosis: a review with presentation of ten new cases. Acta Paediatr Scand 1975;64:362–8.

19. Carlsson G, Fasth A. Infantile genetic agranulocytosis, morbus Kostmann: presentation of six cases from the original "Kostmann family" and a review. Acta Paediatr 2001;90(7):757–64.

20. Horwitz M, Li F-Q, Albani D, et al. Leukemia in severe congenital neutropenia: defective proteolysis suggests new pathways to malignancy and opportunities for therapy. Cancer Invest 2003;21:577–85.

21. Klein C. Genetic defects in severe congenital neutropenia: emerging insights into life and death of human neutrophil granulocytes. Annu Rev Immunol 2011;29:399–413.

22. Donadieu J, Fenneteau O, Beaupain B, et al. Congenital neutropenia: diagnosis, molecular bases and patient management. Orphanet J Rare Dis 2011;6:26.

23. Carlsson G, van't Hooft I, Melin M, et al. Central nervous system involvement in severe congenital neutropenia: neurological and neuropsychological abnormalities associated with specific HAX1 mutations. J Intern Med 2008;264(4): 388–400.

24. Boztug K, Appaswamy G, Ashikov A, et al. A syndrome with congenital neutropenia and mutations in G6PC3. N Engl J Med 2009;360(1):32–43.

25. Person RE, Li FQ, Duan Z, et al. Mutations in proto-oncogene GFI1 cause human neutropenia and target ELA2. Nat Genet 2003;34(3):308–12.

26. Armistead PM, Wieder E, Akande O, et al. Cyclic neutropenia associated with T cell immunity to granulocyte proteases and a double de novo mutation in GFI1, a transcriptional regulator of ELANE. Br J Haematol 2010;150(6):716–9.

27. Takahashi H, Nukiwa T, Basset P, et al. Myelomonocytic cell lineage expression of the neutrophil elastase gene. J Biol Chem 1988;263(5):2543–7.

28. Kim YM, Haghighat L, Spiekerkoetter E, et al. Neutrophil elastase is produced by pulmonary artery smooth muscle cells and is linked to neointimal lesions. Am J Pathol 2011;179(3):1560–72.

29. Donadieu J, Leblanc T, Bader Meunier B, et al. Analysis of risk factors for mye-lodysplasias, leukemias and death from infection among patients with congenital neutropenia. Experience of the French Severe Chronic Neutropenia Study Group. Haematologica 2005;90(1):45–53.
30. Rosenberg PS, Zeidler C, Bolyard AA, et al. Stable long-term risk of leukaemia in patients with severe congenital neutropenia maintained on G-CSF therapy. Br J Haematol 2010;150(2):196–9.
31. Carlsson G, Fasth A, Berglof E, et al. Incidence of severe congenital neutropenia in Sweden and risk of evolution to myelodysplastic syndrome/leukaemia. Br J Haematol 2012;158(3):363–9.
32. Freedman MH, Bonilla MA, Fier C, et al. Myelodysplasia syndrome and acute myeloid leukemia in patients with congenital neutropenia receiving G-CSF therapy. Blood 2000;96(2):429–36.
33. Donadieu J, Fenneteau O, Beaupain B, et al. Classification and risk factors of hematological complications in a French national cohort of 102 patients with Shwachman-Diamond syndrome. Haematologica 2012;97(9):1312–9.
34. Dong F, Brynes RK, Tidow N, et al. Mutations in the gene for the granulocyte colony-stimulating-factor receptor in patients with acute myeloid leukemia preceded by severe congenital neutropenia. N Engl J Med 1995;333(8):487–93.
35. Sinha S, Zhu QS, Romero G, et al. Deletional mutation of the external domain of the human granulocyte colony-stimulating factor receptor in a patient with severe chronic neutropenia refractory to granulocyte colony-stimulating factor. J Pediatr Hematol Oncol 2003;25(10):791–6.
36. Liu F, Kunter G, Krem MM, et al. Csf3r mutations in mice confer a strong clonal HSC advantage via activation of Stat5. J Clin Invest 2008;118(3):946–55.
37. Lightsey AL, Parmley RT, Marsh WL Jr, et al. Severe congenital neutropenia with unique features of dysgranulopoiesis. Am J Hematol 1985;18(1):59–71.
38. Putsep K, Carlsson G, Boman HG, et al. Deficiency of antibacterial peptides in patients with morbus Kostmann: an observation study. Lancet 2002;360(9340): 1144–9.
39. Kawaguchi H, Kobayashi M, Nakamura K, et al. Dysregulation of transcriptions in primary granule constituents during myeloid proliferation and differentiation in patients with severe congenital neutropenia. J Leukoc Biol 2003;73(2):225–34.
40. Sera Y, Kawaguchi H, Nakamura K, et al. A comparison of the defective granulopoiesis in childhood cyclic neutropenia and in severe congenital neutropenia. Haematologica 2005;90(8):1032–41.
41. Donini M, Fontana S, Savoldi G, et al. G-CSF treatment of severe congenital neutropenia reverses neutropenia but does not correct the underlying functional deficiency of the neutrophil in defending against microorganisms. Blood 2007; 109(11):4716–23.
42. Habscheid W, Bernhardt C, Sold M, et al. Atraumatic Clostridium septicum infection in granulocytopenia. Dtsch Med Wochenschr 1991;116(49):1862–6 [in German].
43. van Winkelhoff AJ, Schouten-van Meeteren AY, Baart JA, et al. Microbiology of destructive periodontal disease in adolescent patients with congenital neutropenia. A report of 3 cases. J Clin Periodontol 2000;27(11):793–8.
44. Dick EP, Prince LR, Sabroe I. Ex vivo-expanded bone marrow CD34+ derived neutrophils have limited bactericidal ability. Stem Cells 2008;26(10):2552–63.
45. Yakisan E, Schirg E, Zeidler C, et al. High incidence of significant bone loss in patients with severe congenital neutropenia (Kostmann's syndrome). J Pediatr 1997;131(4):592–7.

46. Boechat MI, Gormley LS, O'Laughlin BJ. Thickened cortical bones in congenital neutropenia. Pediatr Radiol 1987;17(2):124–6.
47. Fewtrell MS, Kinsey SE, Williams DM, et al. Bone mineralization and turnover in children with congenital neutropenia, and its relationship to treatment with recombinant human granulocyte-colony stimulating factor. Br J Haematol 1997;97(4):734–6.
48. Bishop NJ, Williams DM, Compston JC, et al. Osteoporosis in severe congenital neutropenia treated with granulocyte colony-stimulating factor. Br J Haematol 1995;89(4):927–8.
49. Sekhar RV, Culbert S, Hoots WK, et al. Severe osteopenia in a young boy with Kostmann's congenital neutropenia treated with granulocyte colony-stimulating factor: suggested therapeutic approach. Pediatrics 2001;108(3):E54.
50. Hirbe AC, Uluckan O, Morgan EA, et al. Granulocyte colony-stimulating factor enhances bone tumor growth in mice in an osteoclast-dependent manner. Blood 2007;109(8):3424–31.
51. Christopher MJ, Link DC. Granulocyte colony-stimulating factor induces osteoblast apoptosis and inhibits osteoblast differentiation. J Bone Miner Res 2008; 23(11):1765–74.
52. Horwitz M, Benson KF, Person RE, et al. Mutations in ELA2, encoding neutrophil elastase, definea 21-day biological clock in cyclic haematopoiesis. Nat Genet 1999;23(4):433–6.
53. Korkmaz B, Horwitz MS, Jenne DE, et al. Neutrophil elastase, proteinase 3, and cathepsin G as therapeutic targets in human diseases. Pharmacol Rev 2010; 62(4):726–59.
54. Dale DC, Person RE, Bolyard AA, et al. Mutations in the gene encoding neutrophil elastase in congenital and cyclic neutropenia. Blood 2000;96(7):2317–22.
55. Germeshausen M, Zeidler C, Stuhrmann M, et al. Digenic mutations in severe congenital neutropenia. Haematologica 2010;95(7):1207–10.
56. Xia J, Bolyard AA, Rodger E, et al. Prevalence of mutations in ELANE, GFI1, HAX1, SBDS, WAS and G6PC3 in patients with severe congenital neutropenia. Br J Haematol 2009;147(4):535–42.
57. Lanciotti M, Caridi G, Rosano C, et al. Severe congenital neutropenia: a negative synergistic effect of multiple mutations of ELANE (ELA2) gene. Br J Haematol 2009;146(5):578–80.
58. Bellanne-Chantelot C, Clauin S, Leblanc T, et al. Mutations in the ELA2 gene correlate with more severe expression of neutropenia: a study of 81 patients from the French neutropenia register. Blood 2004;103(11):4119–25.
59. Newburger PE, Pindyck TN, Zhu Z, et al. Cyclic neutropenia and severe congenital neutropenia in patients with a shared ELANE mutation and paternal haplotype: evidence for phenotype determination by modifying genes. Pediatr Blood Cancer 2010;55(2):314–7.
60. Boxer LA, Stein S, Buckley D, et al. Strong evidence for autosomal dominant inheritance of severe congenital neutropenia associated with ELA2 mutations. J Pediatr 2006;148(5):633–6.
61. Klein C, Grudzien M, Appaswamy G, et al. HAX1 deficiency causes autosomal recessive severe congenital neutropenia (Kostmann disease). Nat Genet 2007; 39(1):86–92.
62. Carlsson G, Aprikyan AA, Ericson KG, et al. Neutrophil elastase and granulocyte colony-stimulating factor receptor mutation analyses and leukemia evolution in severe congenital neutropenia patients belonging to the original Kostmann family in northern Sweden. Haematologica 2006;91(5):589–95.

63. Salipante SJ, Benson KF, Luty J, et al. Double de novo mutations of ELA2 in cyclic and severe congenital neutropenia. Hum Mutat 2007;28(9):874–81.
64. Goriely A, Wilkie AO. Paternal age effect mutations and selfish spermatogonial selection: causes and consequences for human disease. Am J Hum Genet 2012;90(2):175–200.
65. Zlotogora J. Germ line mosaicism. Hum Genet 1998;102(4):381–6.
66. Ancliff PJ, Gale RE, Hann IM, et al. Paternal mosaicism proves the pathogenic nature of mutations in neutrophil elastase in severe congenital neutropenia. Blood 2001;98:1841a. Available at: http://www.ncbi.nlm.nih.gov/pubmed/12091371.
67. Germeshausen M, Schulze H, Ballmaier M, et al. Mutations in the gene encoding neutrophil elastase (ELA2) are not sufficient to cause the phenotype of congenital neutropenia. Br J Haematol 2001;115:222–4.
68. Malcov M, Reches A, Ben-Yosef D, et al. Resolving a genetic paradox throughout preimplantation genetic diagnosis for autosomal dominant severe congenital neutropenia. Prenat Diagn 2010;30(3):207–11.
69. Benson KF, Horwitz M. Possibility of somatic mosaicism of ELA2 mutation overlooked in an asymptomatic father transmitting severe congenital neutropenia to two offspring. Br J Haematol 2002;118:923.
70. Ancliff PJ, Gale RE, Liesner R, et al. Mutations in the ELA2 gene encoding neutrophil elastase are present in most patients with sporadic severe congenital neutropenia but only in some patients with the familial form of the disease. Blood 2001;98(9):2645–50.
71. Beekman R, Valkhof MG, Sanders MA, et al. Sequential gain of mutations in severe congenital neutropenia progressing to acute myeloid leukemia. Blood 2012;119(22):5071–7.
72. Xia J, Link DC. Severe congenital neutropenia and the unfolded protein response. Curr Opin Hematol 2008;15(1):1–7.
73. Sherry ST, Ward MH, Kholodov M, et al. dbSNP: the NCBI database of genetic variation. Nucleic Acids Res 2001;29(1):308–11.
74. Nagy E, Maquat LE. A rule for termination-codon position within intron-containing genes: when nonsense affects RNA abundance. Trends Biochem Sci 1998;23(6):198–9.
75. Thusberg J, Vihinen M. Bioinformatic analysis of protein structure-function relationships: case study of leukocyte elastase (ELA2) missense mutations. Hum Mutat 2006;27(12):1230–43.
76. Massullo P, Druhan LJ, Bunnell BA, et al. Aberrant subcellular targeting of the G185R neutrophil elastase mutant associated with severe congenital neutropenia induces premature apoptosis of differentiating promyelocytes. Blood 2005;105(9):3397–404.
77. Janoff A, Scherer J. Mediators of inflammation in leukocyte lysosomes. IX. Elastinolytic activity in granules of human polymorphonuclear leukocytes. J Exp Med 1968;128(5):1137–55.
78. Weinrauch Y, Drujan D, Shapiro SD, et al. Neutrophil elastase targets virulence factors of enterobacteria. Nature 2002;417(6884):91–4.
79. Belaaouaj A, Kim KS, Shapiro SD. Degradation of outer membrane protein A in Escherichia coli killing by neutrophil elastase. Science 2000;289(5482):1185–8.
80. Korkmaz B, Hajjar E, Kalupov T, et al. Influence of charge distribution at the active site surface on the substrate specificity of human neutrophil protease 3 and elastase. A kinetic and molecular modeling analysis. J Biol Chem 2007;282(3):1989–97.

81. Valenzuela-Fernandez A, Planchenault T, Baleux F, et al. Leukocyte elastase negatively regulates Stromal cell-derived factor-1 (patients with SCN-1)/ CXCR4 binding and functions by amino-terminal processing of patients with SCN-1 and CXCR4. J Biol Chem 2002;277(18):15677–89.

82. Ma Q, Jones D, Borghesani PR, et al. Impaired B-lymphopoiesis, myelopoiesis, and derailed cerebellar neuron migration in CXCR4- and SDF-1-deficient mice. Proc Natl Acad Sci U S A 1998;95(16):9448–53.

83. Hernandez PA, Gorlin RJ, Lukens JN, et al. Mutations in the chemokine receptor gene CXCR4 are associated with WHIM syndrome, a combined immunodeficiency disease. Nat Genet 2003;34(1):70–4.

84. Carter CR, Whitmore KM, Thorpe R. The significance of carbohydrates on G-CSF: differential sensitivity of G-CSFs to human neutrophil elastase degradation. J Leukoc Biol 2003;75:515–22.

85. El Ouriaghli F, Fujiwara H, Melenhorst JJ, et al. Neutrophil elastase enzymatically antagonizes the in vitro action of G-CSF: implications for the regulation of granulopoiesis. Blood 2003;101(5):1752–8.

86. Hunter MG, Druhan LJ, Avalos BR. Proteolytic cleavage of G-CSF and the G-CSFR by neutrophil elastase induces growth inhibition and decreased G-CSFR surface expression: implications for myelopoiesis. Blood 2002;100:244a. Available at: http://www.ncbi.nlm.nih.gov/pubmed/14587040.

87. Gullberg U, Bengtsson N, Bulow E, et al. Processing and targeting of granule proteins in human neutrophils. J Immunol Methods 1999;232(1–2):201–10.

88. Adkison AM, Raptis SZ, Kelley DG, et al. Dipeptidyl peptidase I activates neutrophil-derived serine proteases and regulates the development of acute experimental arthritis. J Clin Invest 2002;109(3):363–71.

89. Neurath H. Evolution of proteolytic enzymes. Science 1984;224(4647):350–7.

90. Toomes C, James J, Wood AJ, et al. Loss-of-function mutations in the cathepsin C gene result in periodontal disease and palmoplantar keratosis. Nat Genet 1999;23(4):421–4.

91. Bode W, Meyer E Jr, Powers JC. Human leukocyte and porcine pancreatic elastase: X-ray crystal structures, mechanism, substrate specificity, and mechanism-based inhibitors. Biochemistry 1989;28(5):1951–63.

92. Ortiz PG, Skov BG, Benfeldt E. Alpha1-antitrypsin deficiency-associated panniculitis: case report and review of treatment options. J Eur Acad Dermatol Venereol 2005;19(4):487–90.

93. Bottomley SP. The structural diversity in alpha1-antitrypsin misfolding. EMBO Rep 2011;12(10):983–4.

94. Zeng W, Silverman GA, Remold-O'Donnell E. Structure and sequence of human M/NEI (monocyte/neutrophil elastase inhibitor), an Ov-serpin family gene. Gene 1998;213(1–2):179–87.

95. Ye S, Goldsmith EJ. Serpins and other covalent protease inhibitors. Curr Opin Struct Biol 2001;11(6):740–5.

96. Moreau T, Baranger K, Dade S, et al. Multifaceted roles of human elafin and secretory leukocyte proteinase inhibitor (SLPI), two serine protease inhibitors of the chelonianin family. Biochimie 2008;90(2):284–95.

97. Doumas S, Kolokotronis A, Stefanopoulos P. Anti-inflammatory and antimicrobial roles of secretory leukocyte protease inhibitor. Infect Immun 2005;73(3): 1271–4.

98. Grenda DS, Johnson SE, Mayer JR, et al. Mice expressing a neutrophil elastase mutation derived from patients with severe congenital neutropenia have normal granulopoiesis. Blood 2002;100(9):3221–8.

99. Chao JR, Parganas E, Boyd K, et al. Hax1-mediated processing of HtrA2 by Parl allows survival of lymphocytes and neurons. Nature 2008;452(7183):98–102.

100. Karsunky H, Zeng H, Schmidt T, et al. Inflammatory reactions and severe neutropenia in mice lacking the transcriptional repressor Gfi1. Nat Genet 2002;30(3):295–300.

101. Hock H, Hamblen MJ, Rooke HM, et al. Intrinsic requirement for zinc finger transcription factor Gfi-1 in neutrophil differentiation. Immunity 2003;18: 109–20.

102. Zarebski A, Velu CS, Baktula AM, et al. The human severe congenital neutropenia-associated Gfi1 N382S mutant blocks murine granulopoiesis through CSF1. Immunity 2008. Available at: http://www.ncbi.nlm.nih.gov/pub med/18328744.

103. Cheung YY, Kim SY, Yiu WH, et al. Impaired neutrophil activity and increased susceptibility to bacterial infection in mice lacking glucose-6-phosphatase-beta. J Clin Invest 2007;117(3):784–93.

104. Smirnova OA. Mathematical model of cyclic kinetics of granulocytopoiesis. Kosm Biol Aviakosm Med 1985;19(1):77–80 [in Russian].

105. Pacheco JM, Traulsen A, Antal T, et al. Cyclic neutropenia in mammals. Am J Hematol 2008;83(12):920–1.

106. Morley A. Cyclic hemopoiesis and feedback control. Blood Cells 1979;5(2): 283–96.

107. Haurie C, Dale DC, Mackey MC. Cyclical neutropenia and other periodic hema-tological disorders: a review of mechanisms and mathematical models. Blood 1998;92(8):2629–40.

108. Horwitz M, Benson KF, Duan Z, et al. Role of neutrophil elastase in bone marrow failure syndromes: molecular genetic revival of the chalone hypothesis. Curr Opin Hematol 2003;10(1):49–54.

109. Rytomaa T. Role of chalone in granulopoiesis. Br J Haematol 1973;24:141–6.

110. Leitch HA, Levy JG. Reversal of camal-mediated alterations of normal and leukemic in-vitro myelopoiesis using inhibitors of proteolytic activity. Leukemia 1994;8(4):605–11.

111. Li FQ, Horwitz M. Characterization of mutant neutrophil elastase in severe congenital neutropenia. J Biol Chem 2001;276:14230–41.

112. Kollner I, Sodeik B, Schreek S, et al. Mutations in neutrophil elastase causing congenital neutropenia lead to cytoplasmic protein accumulation and induction of the unfolded protein response. Blood 2006;108(2):493–500.

113. Aoki Y. Crystallization and characterization of a new protease in mitochondria of bone marrow cells. J Biol Chem 1978;253(6):2026–32.

114. Clark JM, Vaughan DW, Aiken BM, et al. Elastase-like enzymes in human neutro-phils localized by ultrastructural cytochemistry. J Cell Biol 1980;84(1):102–19.

115. Kolkenbrock H, Zimmermann J, Burmester GR, et al. Activation of progelatinase B by membranes of human polymorphonuclear granulocytes. Biol Chem 2000; 381(1):49–55.

116. Owen CA, Campbell MA, Sannes PL, et al. Cell surface-bound elastase and cathepsin G on human neutrophils: a novel, non-oxidative mechanism by which neutrophils focus and preserve catalytic activity of serine proteinases. J Cell Biol 1995;131(3):775–89.

117. Lane AA, Ley TJ. Neutrophil elastase is important for PML-retinoic acid receptor alpha activities in early myeloid cells. Mol Cell Biol 2005;25(1):23–33.

118. Belmokhtar CA, Torriglia A, Counis MF, et al. Nuclear translocation of a leukocyte elastase inhibitor/elastase complex during staurosporine-induced apoptosis:

role in the generation of nuclear L-DNase II activity. Exp Cell Res 2000;254(1): 99–109.

119. Nakagami Y, Ito M, Hara T, et al. Loss of TRF2 by radiation-induced apoptosis in HL60 cells. Radiat Med 2002;20(3):121–9.

120. Torriglia A, Perani P, Brossas JY, et al. L-DNase II, a molecule that links proteases and endonucleases in apoptosis, derives from the ubiquitous serpin leukocyte elastase inhibitor. Mol Cell Biol 1998;18(6):3612–9.

121. Papayannopoulos V, Metzler KD, Hakkim A, et al. Neutrophil elastase and myeloperoxidase regulate the formation of neutrophil extracellular traps. J Cell Biol 2010;191(3):677–91.

122. Salipante SJ, Rojas ME, Korkmaz B, et al. Contributions to neutropenia from PFAAP5 (N4BP2L2), a novel protein mediating transcriptional repressor cooperation between Gfi1 and neutrophil elastase. Mol Cell Biol 2009;29(16):4394–405.

123. Benson KF, Li FQ, Person RE, et al. Mutations associated with neutropenia in dogs and humans disrupt intracellular transport of neutrophil elastase. Nat Genet 2003;35(1):90–6.

124. Campbell EJ, Owen CA. The sulfate groups of chondroitin sulfate- and heparan sulfate-containing proteoglycans in neutrophil plasma membranes are novel binding sites for human leukocyte elastase and cathepsin G. J Biol Chem 2007;282(19):14645–54.

125. Lothrop CD Jr, Coulson PA, Nolan HL, et al. Cyclic hormonogenesis in gray collie dogs: interactions of hematopoietic and endocrine systems. Endocrinology 1987;120(3):1027–32.

126. Horwitz M, Benson KF, Duan Z, et al. Hereditary neutropenia: dogs explain human neutrophil elastase mutations. Trends Mol Med, in press. Available at: http://www.ncbi.nlm.nih.gov/pubmed/15059607.

127. Chiang PW, Spector E, Thomas M, et al. Novel mutation causing Hermansky-Pudlak syndrome type 2. Pediatr Blood Cancer 2010;55(7):1438.

128. Li W, Feng Y, Hao C, et al. The BLOC interactomes form a network in endosomal transport. J Genet Genomics 2007;34(8):669–82.

129. Richmond B, Huizing M, Knapp J, et al. Melanocytes derived from patients with Hermansky-Pudlak syndrome types 1, 2, and 3 have distinct defects in cargo trafficking. J Invest Dermatol 2005;124(2):420–7.

130. Meng R, Bridgman R, Toivio-Kinnucan M, et al. Neutrophil elastase-processing defect in cyclic hematopoietic dogs. Exp Hematol 2010;38(2):104–15.

131. Introne W, Boissy RE, Gahl WA. Clinical, molecular, and cell biological aspects of Chediak-Higashi syndrome. Mol Genet Metab 1999;68(2):283–303.

132. Barbosa MD, Nguyen QA, Tchernev VT, et al. Identification of the homologous beige and Chediak-Higashi syndrome genes. Nature 1996;382(6588):262–5.

133. Cavarra E, Martorana PA, Cortese S, et al. Neutrophils in beige mice secrete normal amounts of cathepsin G and a 46 kDa latent form of elastase that can be activated extracellularly by proteolytic activity. Biol Chem 1997;378(5): 417–23.

134. Gallin JI, Bujak JS, Patten E, et al. Granulocyte function in the Chediak-Higashi syndrome of mice. Blood 1974;43(2):201–6.

135. Kramer JW, Davis WC, Prieur DJ. The Chediak-Higashi syndrome of cats. Lab Invest 1977;36(5):554–62.

136. Prieur DJ, Collier LL. Neutropenia in cats with the Chediak-Higashi syndrome. Can J Vet Res 1987;51(3):407–8.

137. Duan Z, Horwitz M. Gfi-1 takes center stage in hematopoietic stem cells. Trends Mol Med 2005;11(2):49–52.

138. Duan Z, Horwitz M. Targets of the transcriptional repressor oncoprotein Gfi-1. Proc Natl Acad Sci U S A 2003;100(10):5932–7.

139. Grenda DS, Murakami M, Ghatak J, et al. Mutations of the ELA2 gene found in patients with severe congenital neutropenia induce the unfolded protein response and cellular apoptosis. Blood 2007;110(13):4179–87.

140. Nanua S, Murakami M, Xia J, et al. Activation of the unfolded protein response is associated with impaired granulopoiesis in transgenic mice expressing mutant Elane. Blood 2011;117(13):3539–47.

141. Delepine M, Nicolino M, Barrett T, et al. EIF2AK3, encoding translation initiation factor 2-alpha kinase 3, is mutated in patients with Wolcott-Rallison syndrome. Nat Genet 2000;25(4):406–9.

142. Senee V, Vattem KM, Delepine M, et al. Wolcott-Rallison syndrome: clinical, genetic, and functional study of EIF2AK3 mutations and suggestion of genetic heterogeneity. Diabetes 2004;53(7):1876–83.

143. Demo SD, Kirk CJ, Aujay MA, et al. Antitumor activity of PR-171, a novel irreversible inhibitor of the proteasome. Cancer Res 2007;67(13):6383–91.

144. Parmley RT, Presbury GJ, Wang WC, et al. Cyclic ultrastructural abnormalities in human cyclic neutropenia. Am J Pathol 1984;116(2):279–88.

Genetics and Pathophysiology of Severe Congenital Neutropenia Syndromes Unrelated to Neutrophil Elastase

Kaan Boztug, MD[a], Christoph Klein, MD, PhD[b],*

KEYWORDS

• Genetics • Pathophysiology • Congenital neutropenia

KEY POINTS

- Considerable progress has been made in recent years in understanding of the genetic basis for congenital neutropenia syndromes.
- With the advent of high-throughput genomic analyzing technologies, the underlying genetic causes of other congenital neutropenia syndromes are expected to be resolved in the near future.
- This knowledge will provide the foundation for genotype-phenotype correlations for infection susceptibility, response to therapy, and risk of malignant transformation, enabling optimal care for individual patients depending on their molecular pathophysiology.
- It is hoped that these investigations will enable the development of tailored molecular therapies to specifically correct the aberrant signaling cascades.

INTRODUCTION

Congenital neutropenia represents a heterogeneous group of inherited disorders with the common denominator of persistent and genetically determined paucity of neutrophil granulocytes in the peripheral blood. Neutropenia is termed mild when absolute neutrophil counts (ANCs) range from 1.0 to 1.5 × 10^9/L, moderate with ANCs from 0.5 to 1.0 × 10^9/L, and severe when ANCs are less than 0.5 × 10^9/L.

This work was partially supported by the START Program of the Austrian Science Fund (FWF): [Y595B13] to K.B. and grants from the European Research Council (ERC-Advanced) and the BMBF (E-RARE, PIDNET) to C.K.

a Department of Pediatrics and Adolescent Medicine, CeMM Research Center for Molecular Medicine of the Austrian Academy of Sciences, Medical University of Vienna, Lazarettgasse 14 AKH BT 25.3, A-1090 Vienna, Austria; b Department of Pediatrics, Dr von Hauner Children's Hospital, University Children's Hospital, Ludwig Maximilians University, Lindwurmstraße 4, D-80337 Munich, Germany
* Corresponding author.
E-mail address: christoph.klein@med.uni-muenchen.de

Hematol Oncol Clin N Am 27 (2013) 43–60
http://dx.doi.org/10.1016/j.hoc.2012.11.004
0889-8588/13/$ – see front matter © 2013 Elsevier Inc. All rights reserved.

Congenital neutropenia has to be distinguished from autoimmune neutropenias (usually self-limiting and not causing severe bacterial infections) and benign ethnic neutropenia (prevalent in the Middle East and Africa, not predisposing to infections). By contrast, congenital neutropenia leads to recurrent and severe bacterial (and sometimes fungal) infections.[1,2] The classic phenotype of autosomal recessive severe congenital neutropenia (SCN) was described by the Swedish pediatrician Rolf Kostmann[1,3] almost 60 years ago.

In the past, the genetic basis for several mendelian diseases with congenital neutropenia were elucidated and improved understanding of the molecular processes underlying this group of disorders (**Table 1**). In the United States and Europe, most patients with SCN have either sporadic or autosomal dominance inheritance patterns and bear monoallelic mutations in the *neutrophil elastase* (*ELANE*) gene (see the article by Horwitz and colleagues elsewhere in this issue for further exploration of this topic). The molecular basis for autosomal recessive SCN is heterogeneous. The classic variant, originally described by Rolf Kostmann,[1,3] is caused by mutations in the gene encoding for the mitochondrial protein HS1-associated protein (HAX1). In Europe, mutations in *HAX1* seem to be more common than in the United States and account for up to 15% to 20% of cases[4] of SCN (European Severe Chronic Neutropenia International Registry, unpublished data). Biallelic mutations in the glucose-6-phosphatase catalytic subunit 3 (*G6PC3*) gene cause a complex disorder associating congenital neutropenia and various developmental aberrations such as congenital heart defects, urogenital malformations, and facial dysmorphy. Mutations in the *GFI1* gene or activating mutations in the Wiskott-Aldrich syndrome (*WAS*) gene represent rare molecular causes of SCN. The relative frequency of these distinct gene defects among patients with SCN differs depending on ethnicity. In particular, in populations with a high degree of consanguinity, autosomal recessive variants of SCN are more prevalent than mutations in *ELANE*. Despite recent progress in the field, in around one-third of patients with SCN, no pathogenic mutations can be identified.

This article discusses some of the most recent findings and discusses their implications for molecular understanding of neutrophil biology.[5,6]

ETHNIC NEUTROPENIA

The most common genetically determined variant associated with congenital neutropenia occurs in areas of the world where *Plasmodium vivax* is endemic, such as Africa and some regions in the Middle East: a polymorphism in *DARC* (Duffy null) is associated with ethnic neutropenia[7] and an increased risk of HIV infection on exposure,[8] although it confers protection against *P vivax* infection.[9,10] Ethnic neutropenia was described decades ago without knowledge of its genetic basis.[11,12] In contrast with patients with SCN, ethnic neutropenia is not associated with severe infections.[12] The molecular details of how the *DARC* polymorphism causes neutropenia and why affected individuals rarely show severe infections as expected for neutropenic patients have remained elusive.

HAX1 DEFICIENCY

Since the original description by Rolf Kostmann,[1,3] it was evident that the classic variant of SCN is a disease with an autosomal recessive inheritance pattern. Using a combination of a genome-wide linkage analysis and candidate gene sequencing, a deleterious mutation in *HAX1* was identified in 3 unrelated consanguineous kindreds from Turkey.[4] The frequency of *HAX1* mutations among patients with SCN is approximately 15%,[4] with considerable differences in their ethnic backgrounds. Thus, a higher percentage of patients from Turkey and the Middle East bear *HAX1* mutations, whereas mutations are rarer among the US population.[13] *HAX1* mutations were also discovered in descendants from the original families described by Rolf Kostmann[3] in his sentinel article describing SCN as a novel disease entity more than 60 years ago.[3,4]

A fraction of HAX1-deficient patients show, in addition to congenital neutropenia, neurologic disease manifestations such as cognitive impairment, developmental delay and/or epilepsy. These clinical observations could be associated with a clear genotype-phenotype pattern for 2 known isoforms of *HAX1*: isoforms a and b. Although *HAX1* mutations that affect exclusively isoform a show a phenotype of (isolated) congenital neutropenia, mutations affecting both isoforms are associated with additional neurologic aberrations.[14–16] This view has recently been challenged by other investigators[17] who described 1 patient with a compound heterozygous mutation in HAX1 without neurologic findings. Mice with a targeted deletion of *Hax1* show increased neuronal cell apoptosis and a neurodegenerative disorder.[18] The hematological aberrations of Hax1 deficiency in the murine knockout model comprise lymphopenia, including significant reduction of B cells but no overt neutropenia.[18,19] The reasons for this species-related difference are unclear at present but are reminiscent of other disorders such as ELANE deficiency, in which the respective murine transgenic mouse does not model neutropenia.[20,21] Thus, it is possible that murine neutrophil granulocytes behave differently with respect to resistance and susceptibility to apoptosis compared with human cells (see the article by Schäffer A elsewhere in this issue for more details).

HAX1 is a ubiquitously expressed protein that localizes predominantly to the mitochondria.[4,22] Deficiency of HAX1 in hematopoietic and nonhematopoietic cells leads to destabilization of the mitochondrial membrane potential ($\Delta\psi m$),[4] which explains the increased apoptosis observed in myeloid cells as well as nonhematopoietic cells such as fibroblasts.[4] In this respect, the interaction of HAX1 with PARL (presenelin-associated, rhomboidlike) and Htr2A/Omi[18,23] is intriguing, because activation of this pathway leads to activation of proapoptotic BAX.[18] The antiapoptotic activity of HAX1 may alternatively be mediated through interaction with XIAP (X-linked inhibitor of apoptosis protein) by suppressing its polyubiquitination and thus protecting it from degradation in the proteosome.[24] Another interesting observation with potential implications for the role of HAX1 in regulating apoptosis is that it interacts with phospholamban, a cardiac protein inhibiting SERCA2A, a sarcoplasmic reticulum Ca2+-ATPase.[25] More recently, HAX1 was shown to directly interact with SERCA2A and downregulate its expression, which may modulate endoplasmic reticulum (ER) Ca2+ levels.[26] Taken together, the molecular mechanisms that cause deficiency of HAX1 to lead to increased myeloid cell apoptosis are not yet clear. Nevertheless, it seems that HAX1 is a critical regulator of various cellular processes that are directly or indirectly associated with cell survival or apoptosis.

HAX1 interacts with a large number of other cytosolic proteins, including Gα13,[27] Il1α,[28] the polycystic kidney disease 2 (PKD2) protein,[29] integrin $\alpha v \beta 6$,[30] and bile salt protein.[31] These data suggest a role for HAX1 in intracellular transport and cell migration, and a recent study by Cavnar and colleagues[32] revealed a critical role for HAX1 in regulating neutrophil adhesion and chemotaxis through modulation of RhoA signaling.

A large number of additional interaction partners have been identified to date, highlighting a complex proteomic network of HAX1. Interactions with viral proteins such as Karposi sarcoma–associated herpesvirus K15 protein (KSHV),[33] Epstein-Barr virus

Table 1
Genetic defects causing congenital neutropenia

Disease	Gene Mutated	Inheritance	Hematopoietic Manifestations	Extrahematopoietic Manifestations	Pathophysiologic Mechanism	References
(1) SCN						
ELANE deficiency (SCN1)	ELANE	AD	CN or CyN	—	Activation of the UPR, excessive apoptosis of myeloid cells	21,58,59, 114–116
GFI1 deficiency (SCN2)	GFI1	AD	CN, lymphopenia	—	Defective myeloid cell differentiation	70,71,80, 86–88
HAX1 deficiency (SCN3)	HAX1	AR	CN	Epilepsy, neurologic impairment in some patients	Destabilization of mitochondrial membrane potential, excessive apoptosis of myeloid cells	4,14,15,18
G6PC3 deficiency (SCN4)	G6PC3	AR	CN, thrombocytopenia	Congenital heart defects, facial dysmorphy, increased visibility of superficial veins, urogenital malformations, failure to thrive, endocrine abnormalities, inner ear hearing loss, hyperelasticity of the skin	Impaired intracellular glucose homeostasis, activation of the UPR, excessive apoptosis of myeloid cells	42,51,52,60, 61,65,66
XLN	WAS	XL	CN, lymphopenia, myelodysplasia	—	Enhanced and discoordinated actin polymerization, defective cytokinesis	95–97
(2) Congenital neutropenia: hypopigmentation disorders						
Chédiak-Higashi syndrome	LYST/CHS1	AR	CN, defective NK cell function, lysosomal inclusion bodies in leukocytes, macrophage activation syndrome	Oculocutaneous albinism, neurodegeneration	—	117–119

Disorder	Gene	Inheritance	Hematologic/clinical features	Other features	Mechanism/function	Refs
Hermansky-Pudlak syndrome, type 2	AP3B1	AR	CN, impaired function of T and NK cells	Oculocutaneous albinism	Defective endosomal function	120-124
Griscelli syndrome, type 2	RAB27A	AR	CN, defective cytotoxicity, macrophage activation syndrome	Oculocutaneous albinism	—	125,126
P14/ROBLD3/MAPBPIP deficiency	P14/ROBLD3/MAPBPIP	AR	CN, defective cytotoxicity, growth failure, lymphoid immunodeficiency	Oculocutaneous albinism	Aberrant distribution of late endosomes	127
(3) Complex disorders comprising congenital neutropenia						
AK2 deficiency	AK2	AR	CN, severe lymphopenia (reticular dysgenesis)	Inner ear hearing loss	Aberrant mitochondrial metabolism caused by lack of adenylate kinase 2	128,129
Shwachman-Diamond syndrome	SBDS	AR	CN	Exocrine pancreatic insufficiency, skeletal dysplasia, hepatic and cardiac disease	Mitotic spindle destabilization, genomic instability, enhanced apoptosis	130
WHIM syndrome	CXCR4	AD	CN, myelokathexis, B cell deficiency	Warts, hypogammaglobulinemia, immunodeficiency	Constitutive activating mutations in CXCR4 associated with myelokathexis and lack of neutrophils in peripheral blood	131-133
Poikiloderma with neutropenia	C16ORF57	AR	CN, bone marrow abnormalities	Poikiloderma, increased photosensitivity	Disturbed biogenesis of U6 small nuclear RNA, impaired cell viability	98,103,111
Cartilage-hair hypoplasia	RMRP	AR	CN, immunodeficiency	Hypoplastic hair, skeletal dysplasia	Defective assembly of ribosomes, aberrant cell cycle control and telomere function	134-136

(continued on next page)

Table 1
(continued)

Disease	Gene Mutated	Inheritance	Hematopoietic Manifestations	Extrahematopoietic Manifestations	Pathophysiologic Mechanism	References
CD40L deficiency (HIGM1)	CD40L/CD154	XL	Intermittent CN, combined immunodeficiency including T and B cell deficiency, defective B cell class switch (hyper-IgM syndrome type I)	—	Defective class switch caused by impaired CD40-CD40L interaction, defective T cell priming	137
Barth syndrome	G4.5/TAZ	XL	CN (in most patients)	Cardioskeletal myopathy, growth impairment, carnitine deficiency	Mitochondrial dysfunction, excessive apoptosis in myeloid cells	138,139
Cohen syndrome	VPS13B/COH	AR	Intermittent CN	Psychomotor retardation, skeletal dysplasia, hypotonia	Suspected function of COH in vesicular transport processes	140
Pearson syndrome	Deletion of mitochondrial DNA	mtDNA	CN, bone marrow failure	Exocrine pancreas insufficiency, endocrine abnormalities, neuromuscular degeneration	—	141

Abbreviations: AD, autosomal dominant; AR, autosomal recessive; CN, congenital neutropenia; CyN, cyclic neutropenia; IgM, immunoglobulin M; mtDNA, mitochondrial DNA; NK, natural killer; UPR, unfolded protein response; XL, X-linked recessive.
Modified from Boztug K, Klein C. Novel genetic etiologies of severe congenital neutropenia. Curr Opin Immunol 2009;21(5):472–80; with permission.

(EBV) nuclear antigen 5 (EBNA5)[34] and EBV nuclear antigen leader protein (EBNA-LP),[35] HIV-vpr[36] and HIV-rev,[37] hepatitis C virus core protein,[38] and swine fever virus N-terminal protease[39] collectively suggest that several viruses may have usurped additional functions of HAX1 that have remained elusive to date. More recently, it has been recognized that HAX1 also interacts with the 3'untranslated region sequence of several mRNAs.[40,41] Although the functional significance is not clear, these findings suggest a potential role of HAX1 in posttranscriptional control of mRNA processing, stability, and localization.

G6PC3 DEFICIENCY

A previously unrecognized immunodeficiency syndrome associating SCN and complex developmental aberrations has recently been described, caused by mutations in the glucose-6-phosphatase catalytic subunit 3 (G6PC3) gene.[42] G6PC3 is a member of the glucose-6-phosphatase family, consisting of G6PC1, G6PC2, and G6PC3 (reviewed by Hutton and O'Brien[43]).

G6PC1 is predominantly expressed in liver, gut, and kidney, and G6PC2 is expressed in β cells of the pancreas.[44,45] G6PC3 is ubiquitously expressed.[46] Mutations in G6PC1 cause glycogen storage disease type Ia, and, more recently, polymorphisms in G6PC2 have been associated with alterations in fasting glucose levels,[47–49] implicating a critical role for G6PC2 in controlling system glucose levels, although a murine knockout model of G6pc2 does not show increased incidence or progression of type I diabetes.[50] Mutations in G6PC3 have been observed in all exons of the gene, with partial clustering at exons 1 and 6, respectively, encoding for the N-terminal and C-terminal ends of the gene products. No clear-cut genotype-to-phenotype correlations have been observed,[51] but it is possible that such effects will become more obvious when an even larger cohort of patients is available for systematic phenotypic analysis.

In addition to congenital neutropenia, intermittent or persistent thrombocytopenia is a feature of G6PC3 deficiency.[51] Furthermore, G6PC3-deficient patients usually show extrahematopoietic manifestations such as congenital heart or urogenital defects.[51,52] In a cohort of 28 systematically reviewed patients, congenital heart defects (24/28), unusual visibility of superficial veins (24/28), urogenital malformations (13/28), and facial dysmorphy (18/28) were the most frequent aberrations.[51,52] Deficiency of G6PC3 may rarely manifest clinically by inflammatory bowel disease, a feature shared with glucose-6-phosphate translocase deficiency (authors' own observations, see later discussion).

It has been known for a long time that patients with glycogen storage disease type Ib show a phenotype of congenital neutropenia combined with the typical features of glycogen storage disorder.[53,54] The molecular cause of this disorder was subsequently clarified, when mutations in the SLC37A4 gene encoding the ubiquitously expressed glucose-6-phosphate transporter were found.[55] Similar to G6PC1, G6PC3 is thought to act in a functional complex with G6PT on the membrane of the ER. In line with this model, functional deficiency of the G6PC1/G6PT complex is associated with glycogen storage disease, whereas deficiency of the G6PC3/G6PT complex causes congenital neutropenia (reviewed by Boztug and Klein[56]).

Similar to other genetically defined subforms of congenital neutropenia, including ELANE deficiency and HAX1 deficiency,[4,57] G6PC3-deficient congenital neutropenia is associated with increased apoptosis in peripheral neutrophil granulocytes.[52] In line with aberrant ER physiology, deficiency of G6PC3 is associated with increased apoptosis linked to the activation of the so-called unfolded protein response (UPR),[52] as was also shown for ELANE-deficient congenital neutropenia.[58,59] Studies in the respective murine knockout models have shown activation of the UPR, increased neutrophil apoptosis, and neutropenia in both $G6pc3$-deficient[60] as well as $Slc37a4$-deficient mice.[42]

G6PC3 deficiency has shown the critical importance of glucose homeostasis for neutrophil survival.[52] In G6PC3 deficiency, glucose metabolism in neutrophil granulocytes is markedly disturbed with reduced levels of glucose uptake, glucose-6-phosphate, lactate, and adenosine triphosphate (ATP).[61] Glucose deprivation using 2-dioxyglucose therefore leads to massive apoptosis in neutrophils from healthy controls, whereas other hematopoietic cells such as lymphocytes are less vulnerable.[52] A glucose-sensitive apoptosis pathway involving glycogen synthase kinase 3β and the antiapoptotic Bcl2 molecule Mcl1[62,63] were described previously with Mcl1 as an essential antiapoptotic factor specifically in neutrophils.[64] In G6PC3 deficiency, this pathway is activated,[52] highlighting a nutrient-sensitive pathway of critical importance for survival of neutrophils. In G6PC3-deficient mice, treatment with granulocyte colony-stimulating factor (G-CSF) counteracts reduction of glucose-6-phosphate, lactate, and ATP and excessive apoptosis linked to activation of Akt and Caspase-3,[65] and it is likely that G-CSF treatment has similar effects on human neutrophils from G6PC3-deficient patients. In the corresponding knockout mouse model, monocytes/macrophages also show a functional defect including impaired respiratory burst, chemotaxis, calcium flux, and phagocytosis linked to aberrant glucose metabolism.[66] It is unclear at present whether these effects can also be observed in human G6PC3-deficient monocytes/macrophages.

Aberrant ER metabolism may entail not only a reduced threshold for apoptosis but also, more indirectly, on glycosylation patterns of various target proteins critical for neutrophil function, such as nicotinamide adenine dinucleotide phosphate hydrogen (NADPH) oxidase.[67] As a consequence, G6PC3 deficiency can also be associated with qualitative neutrophil defects.[67] Both quantitative and qualitative features of neutrophil dysfunction can be reversed by recombinant G-CSF therapy (Boztug and Klein, unpublished observation, 2010), a finding similar to the response in murine G6PC3-deficient neutrophils.[65]

From a clinical point of view, most G6PC3-deficient patients respond well to low to moderate dosages of G-CSF with increase in neutrophil counts and decreasing frequency and severity of infections.[51] In a cohort of 28 patients, we have not observed any transformation to myelodysplastic syndrome (MDS)/acute myeloblastic leukemia (AML) to date, suggesting that the risk of leukemogenesis may be lower in G6PC3-deficient SCN compared with other genetic subtypes of SCN.[51] Patients with mutations in ELANE or HAX1 and also some patients with still unknown variants of SCN have a higher risk of developing a clonal hematopoietic disorder such as MDS or AML,[68,69] which shows that delineation of the underlying genetic cause of SCN is of critical relevance for affected patients for long-term surveillance and tailored treatment decisions.

RARE MOLECULAR SUBTYPES OF SCN CAUSED BY MUTATIONS IN GFI1 OR WASP

Growth factor independence-1 (GFI1) is an important transcription factor governing myeloid cell differentiation.[70–72] It acts as a transcriptional repressor, controlling hematopoietic stem cell renewal and differentiation, via interaction with various target genes that include genes critical for myeloid cell differentiation, such as CEBPε and CEBPα[73–75] and HoxA9, Pbx1, and Meis1.[76] Furthermore, GFI1 has been shown to interact with BAX, implicating a role in regulation of apoptosis[77] and microRNAs including miR-21, miR-196b, and miR-96.[78,79] A murine knockout model for Gfi1 deficiency has been studied extensively and has revealed severe neutropenia associated with a differentiation block of myeloid cells.[71,80] Later studies have revealed additional defects in hematopoiesis affecting dendritic cells,[72] B cell differentiation,[81,82] and T helper cell differentiation,[83-85] respectively.

Shortly after the discovery that Gfi1-deficient mice are neutropenic,[71] Person and colleagues[86] identified heterozygous mutations in patients with GFI1 (N382S) SCN. This variant has been shown to act in a dominant-negative fashion.[87] GFI1 mutations have also been identified in a patient with cyclic neutropenia.[88] Both GFI1 and ELANE interact with PFAAP5,[89] providing a potential explanation for the decreased expression of ELANE in GFI1-deficient patients.[86] No PFAAP5 mutations have been reported in patients with SCN to date.

Inactivating mutations in the Wiskott-Aldrich syndrome (WAS) gene causes Wiskott-Aldrich syndrome, an X-linked disorder associating immunodeficiency, eczema, microthrombocytopenia, and bleeding diathesis as well as predisposition to malignant lymphoma.[90,91] The corresponding gene product (WAS protein) is critically involved in actin remodeling, which is important for proper functioning of various subsets of leukocytes such as leukocyte migration/chemotaxis, T cell receptor–mediated signal transduction, and formation of the natural killer cell immunologic synapse (reviewed by Thrasher and Burns[92]). In contrast with loss-of-function mutations in WAS, activating mutations in WAS disable the autoinhibitory state, which usually prevents activation of the C-terminal VCA domain and its interaction with the actin-related protein 2/3 (ARP2/3) complex.[92] Several patients have been reported in whom WAS mutations (such as L270P or I294T) disrupt the autoinhibitory state of WASP and lead to SCN and lmyphopenia.[93-95] Molding and colleagues[96] showed that the WASP I294T variant causes increased and delocalized actin polymerization followed by defective cytokinesis and increased apoptosis. The defective cytokinesis may also underlie the myelodysplasia that has been observed in these patients.[93,96,97] These studies have shed light on the importance of adequate regulation of the cytoskeleton for neutrophil survival. Thus far, it is unknown whether additional genetic defects causing SCN are associated with an aberrant architecture of the cytoskeleton.

CLERICUZIO-TYPE POIKILODERMA WITH NEUTROPENIA

Clericuzio-type poikiloderma with neutropenia (PN) is an autosomal recessive disorder first described in 1991 in 14 Navajo Indians.[98] The major features of the syndrome are poikiloderma (chronic skin disorder characterized by hyperpigmentation, hypopigmentation, and telangiectasia) and neutropenia with concomitant bone marrow abnormalities.[98,99] PN shows overlapping clinical features with another autosomal recessive disorder termed Rothmund-Thomson syndrome (RTS; OMIN #268400),[100,101] but patients with RTS do not usually show neutropenia.[102]

Volpi and colleagues[103] recently identified mutations in C16orf57 as the molecular cause of PN. After this discovery, mutations in this gene were identified in other patients with PN.[104-109] C16orf57 mutations were also found in patients who were previously classified as having RTS,[110] underlining the considerable phenotypical overlap between these 2 syndromes.

C16orf57 is thought to directly interact with SMAD4 proteins, which are interconnected to RECQL4.[103] Mroczek and colleagues[111] were recently able to show that the yeast ortholog of C16orf57, USB1, has a critical role for biogenesis of U6 small nuclear RNA and cell viability. Further studies are needed to shed light on the detailed molecular pathogenesis of this peculiar disorder.

DEFINED SYNDROMES WITH CONGENITAL NEUTROPENIA AND HYPOPIGMENTATION

In addition to the classic Kostmann phenotype of SCN, several disorders combining congenital neutropenia and hypopigmentation have been described and have enabled an understanding of the complex interplay between the lysosome biology in pigmentation and the immune system, respectively (reviewed by Stinchcombe and colleagues[112]). Four defined disorders associating congenital neutropenia and hypopigmentation have been described to date: Chédiak-Higashi syndrome (CHS), Griscelli syndrome type 2 (GS2), Hermansky-Pudlak syndrome type 2 (HPS2), and P14/MAPBPIP/LAMTOR2 deficiency. Neutropenia in HPS2 and P14/MAPBPIP/LAMTOR2 deficiency is constant, whereas neutropenia in CHS and GS2 is not consistently seen. In contrast with SCN, mature neutrophils are found in bone marrow smears from these patients, whereas patients show neutropenia in their peripheral blood counts. These disorders have recently been reviewed in detail.[113]

OUTLOOK

Considerable progress has been made in recent years in understanding the genetic basis for congenital neutropenia syndromes. These studies have enhanced understanding of the physiologic processes governing myelopoiesis and neutrophil function.

With the advent of high-throughput genomic analyzing technologies, it is expected that the underlying genetic causes of other congenital neutropenia syndromes will be resolved in the near future. This knowledge will lay the foundation for genotype-phenotype correlations for infection susceptibility, response to therapy, and risk of malignant transformation, enabling optimal care for individual patients depending on their molecular pathophysiology. These investigations may enable the development of tailored molecular therapies to specifically correct the aberrant signaling cascades.

ACKNOWLEDGMENTS

We are committed to many colleagues sharing clinical information and biological samples. We thank the SCN registries in Germany and France and the international Care-for-Rare Alliance.

REFERENCES

1. Kostmann R. Infantile genetic agranulocytosis; agranulocytosis infantilis hereditaria. Acta Paediatr 1956;45(Suppl 105):1–78.
2. Dale DC, Cottle TE, Fier CJ, et al. Severe chronic neutropenia: treatment and follow-up of patients in the Severe Chronic Neutropenia International Registry. Am J Hematol 2003;72:82–93.
3. Kostmann R. Hereditär reticulos - en ny systemsjukdom. Sv Läkartidningen 1950;47:2861–8.
4. Klein C, Grudzien M, Appaswamy G, et al. Hax1 deficiency causes autosomal recessive severe congenital neutropenia (Kostmann disease). Nat Genet 2007;39:86–92.
5. Carlsson G, Melin M, Dahl N, et al. Kostmann syndrome or infantile genetic agranulocytosis, part two: understanding the underlying genetic defects in severe congenital neutropenia. Acta Paediatr 2007;96(6):813–9.
6. Schäffer AA, Klein C. Genetic heterogeneity in severe congenital neutropenia: how many aberrant pathways can kill a neutrophil? Curr Opin Allergy Clin Immunol 2007;7(6):481–94.

7. Reich D, Nalls MA, Kao WH, et al. Reduced neutrophil count in people of African descent is due to a regulatory variant in the Duffy antigen receptor for chemokines gene. PLoS Genet 2009;5(1):e1000360.

8. Ramsuran V, Kulkarni H, He W, et al. Duffy-null-associated low neutrophil counts influence HIV-1 susceptibility in high-risk South African black women. Clin Infect Dis 2011;52(10):1248–56.

9. Horuk R, Chitnis CE, Darbonne WC, et al. A receptor for the malarial parasite *Plasmodium vivax*: the erythrocyte chemokine receptor. Science 1993; 261(5125):1182–4.

10. Miller LH, Mason SJ, Clyde DF, et al. The resistance factor to *Plasmodium vivax* in blacks. The Duffy-blood-group genotype, FyFy. N Engl J Med 1976;295(6): 302–4.

11. Broun GO Jr, Herbig FK, Hamilton JR. Leukopenia in negroes. N Engl J Med 1966;275(25):1410–3.

12. Haddy TB, Rana SR, Castro O. Benign ethnic neutropenia: what is a normal absolute neutrophil count? J Lab Clin Med 1999;133(1):15–22.

13. Xia J, Bolyard AA, Rodger E, et al. Prevalence of mutations in ELANE, GFI1, HAX1, SBDS, WAS and G6PC3 in patients with severe congenital neutropenia. Br J Haematol 2009;147(4):535–42.

14. Germeshausen M, Grudzien M, Zeidler C, et al. Novel HAX1 mutations in patients with severe congenital neutropenia reveal isoform-dependent genotype-phenotype associations. Blood 2008;111(10):4954–7.

15. Carlsson G, van't Hooft I, Melin M, et al. Central nervous system involvement in severe congenital neutropenia: neurological and neuropsychological abnormalities associated with specific HAX1 mutations. J Intern Med 2008;264(4): 388–400.

16. Boztug K, Ding XQ, Hartmann H, et al. HAX1 mutations causing severe congenital neuropenia and neurological disease lead to cerebral microstructural abnormalities documented by quantitative MRI. Am J Med Genet A 2010;152A(12): 3157–63.

17. Xue SL, Li JL, Zou JY, et al. A novel compound heterozygous HAX1 mutation in a Chinese patient with severe congenital neutropenia and chronic myelomonocytic leukemia transformation but without neurodevelopmental abnormalities. Haematologica 2012;97(2):318–20.

18. Chao JR, Parganas E, Boyd K, et al. Hax1-mediated processing of HtrA2 by Parl allows survival of lymphocytes and neurons. Nature 2008;452(7183):98–102.

19. Peckl-Schmid D, Wolkerstorfer S, Konigsberger S, et al. HAX1 deficiency: impact on lymphopoiesis and B-cell development. Eur J Immunol 2010; 40(11):3161–72.

20. Grenda DS, Johnson SE, Mayer JR, et al. Mice expressing a neutrophil elastase mutation derived from patients with severe congenital neutropenia have normal granulopoiesis. Blood 2002;100(9):3221–8.

21. Nanua S, Murakami M, Xia J, et al. Activation of the unfolded protein response is associated with impaired granulopoiesis in transgenic mice expressing mutant Elane. Blood 2011;117(13):3539–47.

22. Suzuki Y, Demoliere C, Kitamura D, et al. HAX-1, a novel intracellular protein, localized on mitochondria, directly associates with HS1, a substrate of Src family tyrosine kinases. J Immunol 1997;158(6):2736–44.

23. Cilenti L, Soundarapandian MM, Kyriazis GA, et al. Regulation of HAX-1 antiapoptotic protein by Omi/HtrA2 protease during cell death. J Biol Chem 2004; 279(48):50295–301.

24. Kang YJ, Jang M, Park YK, et al. Molecular interaction between HAX-1 and XIAP inhibits apoptosis. Biochem Biophys Res Commun 2010;393(4):794–9.
25. Vafiadaki E, Sanoudou D, Arvanitis DA, et al. Phospholamban interacts with HAX-1, a mitochondrial protein with anti-apoptotic function. J Mol Biol 2007; 367(1):65–79.
26. Vafiadaki E, Arvanitis DA, Pagakis SN, et al. The anti-apoptotic protein HAX-1 interacts with SERCA2 and regulates its protein levels to promote cell survival. Mol Biol Cell 2009;20(1):306–18.
27. Radhika V, Onesime D, Ha JH, et al. Galpha13 stimulates cell migration through cortactin-interacting protein Hax-1. J Biol Chem 2004;279(47):49406–13.
28. Kawaguchi Y, Nishimagi E, Tochimoto A, et al. Intracellular il-1alpha-binding proteins contribute to biological functions of endogenous IL-1alpha in systemic sclerosis fibroblasts. Proc Natl Acad Sci U S A 2006;103(39):14501–6.
29. Gallagher AR, Cedzich A, Gretz N, et al. The polycystic kidney disease protein PKD2 interacts with Hax-1, a protein associated with the actin cytoskeleton. Proc Natl Acad Sci U S A 2000;97(8):4017–22.
30. Ramsay AG, Keppler MD, Jazayeri M, et al. HS1-associated protein X-1 regulates carcinoma cell migration and invasion via clathrin-mediated endocytosis of integrin alphavbeta6. Cancer Res 2007;67(11):5275–84.
31. Ortiz DF, Moseley J, Calderon G, et al. Identification of HAX-1 as a protein that binds bile salt export protein and regulates its abundance in the apical membrane of Madin-Darby canine kidney cells. J Biol Chem 2004;279(31): 32761–70.
32. Cavnar PJ, Berthier E, Beebe DJ, et al. Hax1 regulates neutrophil adhesion and motility through RhoA. J Cell Biol 2011;193(3):465–73.
33. Sharp TV, Wang HW, Koumi A, et al. K15 protein of Kaposi's sarcoma-associated herpesvirus is latently expressed and binds to HAX-1, a protein with antiapoptotic function. J Virol 2002;76(2):802–16.
34. Dufva M, Olsson M, Rymo L. Epstein-Barr virus nuclear antigen 5 interacts with HAX-1, a possible component of the B-cell receptor signalling pathway. J Gen Virol 2001;82(Pt 7):1581–7.
35. Matsuda G, Nakajima K, Kawaguchi Y, et al. Epstein-Barr virus (EBV) nuclear antigen leader protein (EBNA-LP) forms complexes with a cellular anti-apoptosis protein Bcl-2 or its EBV counterpart BHRF1 through HS1-associated protein X-1. Microbiol Immunol 2003;47(1):91–9.
36. Yedavalli VS, Shih HM, Chiang YP, et al. Human immunodeficiency virus type 1 Vpr interacts with antiapoptotic mitochondrial protein HAX-1. J Virol 2005; 79(21):13735–46.
37. Modem S, Reddy TR. An anti-apoptotic protein, Hax-1, inhibits the HIV-1 rev function by altering its sub-cellular localization. J Cell Physiol 2008;214(1):14–9.
38. Banerjee A, Saito K, Meyer K, et al. Hepatitis C virus core protein and cellular protein HAX-1 promote 5-fluorouracil-mediated hepatocyte growth inhibition. J Virol 2009;83(19):9663–71.
39. Johns HL, Doceul V, Everett H, et al. The classical swine fever virus N-terminal protease N(pro) binds to cellular HAX-1. J Gen Virol 2010;91(Pt 11):2677–86.
40. Al-Maghrebi M, Brule H, Padkina M, et al. The 3' untranslated region of human vimentin mRNA interacts with protein complexes containing eEF-1gamma and HAX-1. Nucleic Acids Res 2002;30(23):5017–28.
41. Sarnowska E, Grzybowska EA, Sobczak K, et al. Hairpin structure within the 3'UTR of DNA polymerase beta mRNA acts as a post-transcriptional regulatory element and interacts with Hax-1. Nucleic Acids Res 2007;35(16):5499–510.

42. Kim SY, Jun HS, Mead PA, et al. Neutrophil stress and apoptosis underlie myeloid dysfunction in glycogen storage disease type Ib. Blood 2008; 111(12):5704–11.
43. Hutton JC, O'Brien RM. Glucose-6-phosphatase catalytic subunit gene family. J Biol Chem 2009;284(43):29241–5.
44. Arden SD, Zahn T, Steegers S, et al. Molecular cloning of a pancreatic islet-specific glucose-6-phosphatase catalytic subunit-related protein. Diabetes 1999;48(3):531–42.
45. Martin CC, Bischof LJ, Bergman B, et al. Cloning and characterization of the human and rat islet-specific glucose-6-phosphatase catalytic subunit-related protein (IGRP) genes. J Biol Chem 2001;276(27):25197–207.
46. Guionie O, Clottes E, Stafford K, et al. Identification and characterisation of a new human glucose-6-phosphatase isoform. FEBS Lett 2003;551(1–3): 159–64.
47. Bouatia-Naji N, Rocheleau G, Van Lommel L, et al. A polymorphism within the G6PC2 gene is associated with fasting plasma glucose levels. Science 2008; 320(5879):1085–8.
48. Chen WM, Erdos MR, Jackson AU, et al. Variations in the G6PC2/ABCB11 genomic region are associated with fasting glucose levels. J Clin Invest 2008; 118(7):2620–8.
49. Prokopenko I, Langenberg C, Florez JC, et al. Variants in MTNR1B influence fasting glucose levels. Nat Genet 2009;41(1):77–81.
50. Oeser JK, Parekh VV, Wang Y, et al. Deletion of the G6PC2 gene encoding the islet-specific glucose-6-phosphatase catalytic subunit-related protein does not affect the progression or incidence of type 1 diabetes in NOD/ShiLtJ mice. Diabetes 2011;60(11):2922–7.
51. Boztug K, Rosenberg PS, Dorda M, et al. Extended spectrum of human glucose-6-phosphatase catalytic subunit 3 deficiency: novel genotypes and phenotypic variability in severe congenital neutropenia. J Pediatr 2012;160(4): 679–683.e2.
52. Boztug K, Appaswamy G, Ashikov A, et al. A syndrome with congenital neutropenia and mutations in G6PC3. N Engl J Med 2009;360(1):32–43.
53. Beaudet AL, Anderson DC, Michels VV, et al. Neutropenia and impaired neutrophil migration in type Ib glycogen storage disease. J Pediatr 1980;97(6):906–10.
54. Narisawa K, Tada K, Kuzuya T. Neutropenia in type Ib glycogen storage disease. J Pediatr 1981;99(2):334–5.
55. Gerin I, Veiga-da-Cunha M, Achouri Y, et al. Sequence of a putative glucose 6-phosphate translocase, mutated in glycogen storage disease type Ib. FEBS Lett 1997;419(2–3):235–8.
56. Boztug K, Klein C. Novel genetic etiologies of severe congenital neutropenia. Curr Opin Immunol 2009;21(5):472–80.
57. Carlsson G, Aprikyan AA, Tehranchi R, et al. Kostmann syndrome: severe congenital neutropenia associated with defective expression of Bcl-2, constitutive mitochondrial release of cytochrome c, and excessive apoptosis of myeloid progenitor cells. Blood 2004;103(9):3355–61.
58. Grenda DS, Murakami M, Ghatak J, et al. Mutations of the ELA2 gene found in patients with severe congenital neutropenia induce the unfolded protein response and cellular apoptosis. Blood 2007;110(13):4179–87.
59. Köllner I, Sodeik B, Schreek S, et al. Mutations in neutrophil elastase causing congenital neutropenia lead to cytoplasmic protein accumulation and induction of the unfolded protein response. Blood 2006;108(2):493–500.

60. Cheung YY, Kim SY, Yiu WH, et al. Impaired neutrophil activity and increased susceptibility to bacterial infection in mice lacking glucose-6-phosphatase-beta. J Clin Invest 2007;117(3):784–93.

61. Jun HS, Lee YM, Cheung YY, et al. Lack of glucose recycling between endoplasmic reticulum and cytoplasm underlies cellular dysfunction in glucose-6-phosphatase-beta-deficient neutrophils in a congenital neutropenia syndrome. Blood 2010;116(15):2783–92.

62. Maurer U, Charvet C, Wagman AS, et al. Glycogen synthase kinase-3 regulates mitochondrial outer membrane permeabilization and apoptosis by destabilization of MCL-1. Mol Cell 2006;21(6):749–60.

63. Zhao Y, Altman BJ, Coloff JL, et al. Glycogen synthase kinase 3alpha and 3beta mediate a glucose-sensitive antiapoptotic signaling pathway to stabilize Mcl-1. Mol Cell Biol 2007;27(12):4328–39.

64. Dzhagalov I, St John A, He YW. The antiapoptotic protein Mcl-1 is essential for the survival of neutrophils but not macrophages. Blood 2007;109(4):1620–6.

65. Jun HS, Lee YM, Song KD, et al. G-CSF improves murine G6PC3-deficient neutrophil function by modulating apoptosis and energy homeostasis. Blood 2011;117(14):3881–92.

66. Jun HS, Cheung YY, Lee YM, et al. Glucose-6-phosphatase-beta, implicated in a congenital neutropenia syndrome, is essential for macrophage energy homeostasis and functionality. Blood 2012;119(17):4047–55.

67. Hayee B, Antonopoulos A, Murphy EJ, et al. G6PC3 mutations are associated with a major defect of glycosylation: a novel mechanism for neutrophil dysfunction. Glycobiology 2011;21(7):914–24.

68. Rosenberg PS, Alter BP, Bolyard AA, et al. The incidence of leukemia and mortality from sepsis in patients with severe congenital neutropenia receiving long-term G-CSF therapy. Blood 2006;107(12):4628–35.

69. Rosenberg PS, Alter BP, Link DC, et al. Neutrophil elastase mutations and risk of leukaemia in severe congenital neutropenia. Br J Haematol 2008;140(2):210–3.

70. Hock H, Hamblen MJ, Rooke HM, et al. Gfi-1 restricts proliferation and preserves functional integrity of haematopoietic stem cells. Nature 2004;431(7011):1002–7.

71. Karsunky H, Zeng H, Schmidt T, et al. Inflammatory reactions and severe neutropenia in mice lacking the transcriptional repressor Gfi1. Nat Genet 2002;30(3):295–300.

72. Rathinam C, Geffers R, Yucel R, et al. The transcriptional repressor Gfi1 controls STAT3-dependent dendritic cell development and function. Immunity 2005;22(6):717–28.

73. Marteijn JA, van der Meer LT, Van Emst L, et al. Diminished proteasomal degradation results in accumulation of Gfi1 protein in monocytes. Blood 2007;109(1):100–8.

74. Marteijn JA, van der Meer LT, van Emst L, et al. Gfi1 ubiquitination and proteasomal degradation is inhibited by the ubiquitin ligase triad1. Blood 2007;110(9):3128–35.

75. Zhuang D, Qiu Y, Kogan SC, et al. Increased CCAAT enhancer-binding protein epsilon (C/EBPepsilon) expression and premature apoptosis in myeloid cells expressing Gfi-1 N382S mutant associated with severe congenital neutropenia. J Biol Chem 2006;281(16):10745–51.

76. Horman SR, Velu CS, Chaubey A, et al. Gfi1 integrates progenitor versus granulocytic transcriptional programming. Blood 2009;113(22):5466–75.

77. Nakazawa Y, Suzuki M, Manabe N, et al. Cooperative interaction between ETS1 and GFI1 transcription factors in the repression of Bax gene expression. Oncogene 2007;26(24):3541–50.
78. Lewis MA, Quint E, Glazier AM, et al. An ENU-induced mutation of miR-96 associated with progressive hearing loss in mice. Nat Genet 2009;41(5):614–8.
79. Velu CS, Baktula AM, Grimes HL. Gfi1 regulates miR-21 and miR-196b to control myelopoiesis. Blood 2009;113(19):4720–8.
80. Hock H, Hamblen MJ, Rooke HM, et al. Intrinsic requirement for zinc finger transcription factor Gfi-1 in neutrophil differentiation. Immunity 2003;18(1):109–20.
81. Rathinam C, Klein C. Transcriptional repressor Gfi1 integrates cytokine-receptor signals controlling B-cell differentiation. PLoS One 2007;2(3):e306.
82. Rathinam C, Lassmann H, Mengel M, et al. Transcription factor Gfi1 restricts B cell-mediated autoimmunity. J Immunol 2008;181(9):6222–9.
83. Zhu J, Davidson TS, Wei G, et al. Down-regulation of Gfi-1 expression by TGF-beta is important for differentiation of Th17 and CD103+ inducible regulatory T cells. J Exp Med 2009;206(2):329–41.
84. Zhu J, Guo L, Min B, et al. Growth factor independent-1 induced by IL-4 regulates Th2 cell proliferation. Immunity 2002;16(5):733–44.
85. Zhu J, Jankovic D, Grinberg A, et al. Gfi-1 plays an important role in IL-2-mediated Th2 cell expansion. Proc Natl Acad Sci U S A 2006;103(48):18214–9.
86. Person RE, Li FQ, Duan Z, et al. Mutations in proto-oncogene Gfi1 cause human neutropenia and target ELA2. Nat Genet 2003;34(3):308–12.
87. Zarebski A, Velu CS, Baktula AM, et al. Mutations in growth factor independent-1 associated with human neutropenia block murine granulopoiesis through colony stimulating factor-1. Immunity 2008;28(3):370–80.
88. Armistead PM, Wieder E, Akande O, et al. Cyclic neutropenia associated with T cell immunity to granulocyte proteases and a double de novo mutation in Gfi1, a transcriptional regulator of ELANE. Br J Haematol 2010;150(6):716–9.
89. Salipante SJ, Rojas ME, Korkmaz B, et al. Contributions to neutropenia from PFAAP5 (N4BP2L2), a novel protein mediating transcriptional repressor cooperation between Gfi1 and neutrophil elastase. Mol Cell Biol 2009;29(16):4394–405.
90. Notarangelo LD, Miao CH, Ochs HD. Wiskott-Aldrich syndrome. Curr Opin Hematol 2008;15(1):30–6.
91. Ochs HD, Filipovich AH, Veys P, et al. Wiskott-Aldrich syndrome: diagnosis, clinical and laboratory manifestations, and treatment. Biol Blood Marrow Transplant 2009;15(Suppl 1):84–90.
92. Thrasher AJ, Burns SO. WASP: a key immunological multitasker. Nat Rev Immunol 2010;10(3):182–92.
93. Ancliff PJ, Blundell MP, Cory GO, et al. Two novel activating mutations in the Wiskott-Aldrich syndrome protein result in congenital neutropenia. Blood 2006;108(7):2182–9.
94. Beel K, Cotter MM, Blatny J, et al. A large kindred with X-linked neutropenia with an I294T mutation of the Wiskott-Aldrich syndrome gene. Br J Haematol 2009;144(1):120–6.
95. Devriendt K, Kim AS, Mathijs G, et al. Constitutively activating mutation in WASP causes X-linked severe congenital neutropenia. Nat Genet 2001;27(3):313–7.
96. Moulding DA, Blundell MP, Spiller DG, et al. Unregulated actin polymerization by WASP causes defects of mitosis and cytokinesis in X-linked neutropenia. J Exp Med 2007;204(9):2213–24.
97. Westerberg LS, Meelu P, Baptista M, et al. Activating WASP mutations associated with X-linked neutropenia result in enhanced actin polymerization, altered

cytoskeletal responses, and genomic instability in lymphocytes. J Exp Med 2010;207(6):1145–52.

98. Clericuzio C, Hoyme HE, Asse JM. Immune deficient poikiloderma: a new genodermatosis. Am J Hum Genet 1991;49:A661.

99. Erickson RP. Southwestern Athabaskan (Navajo and Apache) genetic diseases. Genet Med 1999;1(4):151–7.

100. Thompson MS. Poikiloderma congenitale: two cases for diagnosis. Proc R Soc Med 1936;29(5):453–5.

101. Vennos EM, Collins M, James WD. Rothmund-Thomson syndrome: review of the world literature. J Am Acad Dermatol 1992;27(5 Pt 1):750–62.

102. Wang LL, Levy ML, Lewis RA, et al. Clinical manifestations in a cohort of 41 Rothmund-Thomson syndrome patients. Am J Med Genet 2001;102(1):11–7.

103. Volpi L, Roversi G, Colombo EA, et al. Targeted next-generation sequencing appoints C16orf57 as Clericuzio-type poikiloderma with neutropenia gene. Am J Hum Genet 2010;86(1):72–6.

104. Arnold AW, Itin PH, Pigors M, et al. Poikiloderma with neutropenia: a novel C16orf57 mutation and clinical diagnostic criteria. Br J Dermatol 2010;163(4): 866–9.

105. Chantorn R, Shwayder T. Poikiloderma with neutropenia: report of three cases including one with calcinosis cutis. Pediatr Dermatol 2012;29(4):463–72.

106. Clericuzio C, Harutyunyan K, Jin W, et al. Identification of a novel C16orf57 mutation in Athabaskan patients with poikiloderma with neutropenia. Am J Med Genet A 2011;155A(2):337–42.

107. Colombo EA, Bazan JF, Negri G, et al. Novel C16orf57 mutations in patients with poikiloderma with neutropenia: bioinformatic analysis of the protein and predicted effects of all reported mutations. Orphanet J Rare Dis 2012;7:7.

108. Concolino D, Roversi G, Muzzi GL, et al. Clericuzio-type poikiloderma with neutropenia syndrome in three sibs with mutations in the C16orf57 gene: delineation of the phenotype. Am J Med Genet A 2010;152A(10):2588–94.

109. Tanaka A, Morice-Picard F, Lacombe D, et al. Identification of a homozygous deletion mutation in C16orf57 in a family with Clericuzio-type poikiloderma with neutropenia. Am J Med Genet A 2010;152A(6):1347–8.

110. Walne AJ, Vulliamy T, Beswick R, et al. Mutations in C16orf57 and normal-length telomeres unify a subset of patients with dyskeratosis congenita, poikiloderma with neutropenia and Rothmund-Thomson syndrome. Hum Mol Genet 2010; 19(22):4453–61.

111. Mroczek S, Krwawicz J, Kutner J, et al. C16orf57, a gene mutated in poikiloderma with neutropenia, encodes a putative phosphodiesterase responsible for the U6 snRNA 3' end modification. Genes Dev 2012;26(17):1911–25.

112. Stinchcombe J, Bossi G, Griffiths GM. Linking albinism and immunity: the secrets of secretory lysosomes. Science 2004;305:55–9.

113. Boztug K, Welte K, Zeidler C, et al. Congenital neutropenia syndromes. Immunol Allergy Clin North Am 2008;28(2):259–75, vii–viii.

114. Dale DC, Person RE, Bolyard AA, et al. Mutations in the gene encoding neutrophil elastase in congenital and cyclic neutropenia. Blood 2000;96(7): 2317–22.

115. Horwitz M, Benson KF, Person RE, et al. Mutations in ELA2, encoding neutrophil elastase, define a 21-day biological clock in cyclic haematopoiesis. Nat Genet 1999;23(4):433–6.

116. Horwitz MS, Duan Z, Korkmaz B, et al. Neutrophil elastase in cyclic and severe congenital neutropenia. Blood 2007;109(5):1817–24.

117. Barbosa MD, Nguyen QA, Tchernev VT, et al. Identification of the homologous beige and Chediak-Higashi syndrome genes. Nature 1996;382:262–5.
118. Nagle DL, Karim MA, Woolf EA, et al. Identification and mutation analysis of the complete gene for Chediak-Higashi syndrome. Nat Genet 1996;14(3):307–11.
119. Perou CM, Moore KJ, Nagle DL, et al. Identification of the murine beige gene by YAC complementation and positional cloning. Nat Genet 1996;13(3):303–8.
120. Clark RH, Stinchcombe JC, Day A, et al. Adaptor protein 3-dependent microtubule-mediated movement of lytic granules to the immunological synapse. Nat Immunol 2003;4(11):1111–20.
121. Dell'Angelica EC, Shotelersuk V, Aguilar RC, et al. Altered trafficking of lysosomal proteins in Hermansky-Pudlak syndrome due to mutations in the beta 3A subunit of the AP-3 adaptor. Mol Cell 1999;3(1):11–21.
122. Enders A, Zieger B, Schwarz K, et al. Lethal hemophagocytic lymphohistiocytosis in Hermansky-Pudlak syndrome type II. Blood 2006;108(1):81–7.
123. Jung J, Bohn G, Allroth A, et al. Identification of a homozygous deletion in the AP3B1 gene causing Hermansky-Pudlak syndrome, type 2. Blood 2006; 108(1):362–9.
124. Fontana S, Parolini S, Vermi W, et al. Innate immunity defects in Hermansky-Pudlak type 2 syndrome. Blood 2006;107(12):4857–64.
125. Menasche G, Feldmann J, Houdusse A, et al. Biochemical and functional characterization of Rab27a mutations occurring in Griscelli syndrome patients. Blood 2003;101(7):2736–42.
126. Menasche G, Pastural E, Feldmann J, et al. Mutations in RAB27A cause Griscelli syndrome associated with haemophagocytic syndrome. Nat Genet 2000;25(2): 173–6.
127. Bohn G, Allroth A, Brandes G, et al. A novel human primary immunodeficiency syndrome caused by deficiency of the endosomal adaptor protein p14. Nat Med 2006;13:38–45.
128. Lagresle-Peyrou C, Six EM, Picard C, et al. Human adenylate kinase 2 deficiency causes a profound hematopoietic defect associated with sensorineural deafness. Nat Genet 2009;41(1):106–11.
129. Pannicke U, Honig M, Hess I, et al. Reticular dysgenesis (aleukocytosis) is caused by mutations in the gene encoding mitochondrial adenylate kinase 2. Nat Genet 2009;41(1):101–5.
130. Boocock GR, Morrison JA, Popovic M, et al. Mutations in SBDS are associated with Shwachman-Diamond syndrome. Nat Genet 2003;33(1):97–101.
131. Dale DC, Bolyard AA, Kelley ML, et al. The CXCR4 antagonist plerixafor is a potential therapy for myelokathexis, WHIM syndrome. Blood 2011;118(18): 4963–6.
132. Hernandez PA, Gorlin RJ, Lukens JN, et al. Mutations in the chemokine receptor gene CXCR4 are associated with WHIM syndrome, a combined immunodeficiency disease. Nat Genet 2003;34(1):70–4.
133. McDermott DH, Liu Q, Ulrick J, et al. The CXCR4 antagonist plerixafor corrects panleukopenia in patients with WHIM syndrome. Blood 2011; 118(18):4957–62.
134. Bordon V, Gennery AR, Slatter MA, et al. Clinical and immunologic outcome of patients with cartilage hair hypoplasia after hematopoietic stem cell transplantation. Blood 2010;116(1):27–35.
135. de la Fuente MA, Recher M, Rider NL, et al. Reduced thymic output, cell cycle abnormalities, and increased apoptosis of T lymphocytes in patients with cartilage-hair hypoplasia. J Allergy Clin Immunol 2011;128(1):139–46.

136. Ridanpaa M, van Eenennaam H, Pelin K, et al. Mutations in the RNA component of RNase MRP cause a pleiotropic human disease, cartilage-hair hypoplasia. Cell 2001;104(2):195–203.
137. Winkelstein JA, Marino MC, Ochs H, et al. The X-linked hyper-IgM syndrome: clinical and immunologic features of 79 patients. Medicine 2003;82:373–84.
138. Barth PG, Scholte JA, Berden JA, et al. An X-linked mitochondrial disease affecting cardiac muscle, skeletal muscle and neutrophil leukocyte. J Neurol Sci 1983;62:327–55.
139. Barth PG, Valianpour F, Bowen VM, et al. X-linked cardioskeletal myopathy and neutropenia (Barth syndrome): an update. Am J Med Genet 2004;126A:349–54.
140. Kolehmainen J, Black GC, Saarinen A, et al. Cohen syndrome is caused by mutations in a novel gene, COH1, encoding a transmembrane protein with a presumed role in vesicle-mediated sorting and intracellular protein transport. Am J Hum Genet 2003;72:1359–62.
141. Pearson HA, Lobel JS, Kocoshis SA, et al. A new syndrome of refractory sideroblastic anemia with vacuolization of marrow precursors and exocrine pancreatic dysfunction. J Pediatr 1979;95:976–84.

Granulocyte Colony-Stimulating Factor Receptor Signaling

Implications for G-CSF Responses and Leukemic Progression in Severe Congenital Neutropenia

Ivo P. Touw, PhD[a],*, Karishma Palande, PhD[b],
Renée Beekman, MD[a]

KEYWORDS

- G-CSF • G-CSF receptor • Signal transduction • Severe congenital neutropenia
- Leukemia

KEY POINTS

- Although granulocyte colony-stimulating factor (G-CSF) has been routinely used for more than 2 decades to treat various types of severe congenital neutropenia (SCN), the underlying mechanisms of G-CSF hyporesponsiveness or nonresponsiveness have remained largely elusive.
- A thorough understanding of the biology of G-CSF receptor (G-CSFR) activation and signaling function in relation to endosomal and lysosomal trafficking will be useful in identifying compounds that may act synergistically with G-CSF to overcome hyporesponsiveness or nonresponsiveness in SCN.
- It may shed light on how abnormal function of the G-CSFR, caused by mutations that prevent their normal intracellular trafficking, contribute to a premalignant state of hematopoietic stem and progenitor cells.
- Specifically, it remains to be resolved whether G-CSF merely drives the clonal expansion of the "sick" stem cells in SCN or actively contributes to the leukemic process through elevated production of ROS after activation of the truncated G-CSFR, leading to chronic DNA damage, acquisition of additional mutations, and rewiring of signaling and transcription regulatory processes.

GRANULOCYTE COLONY-STIMULATING FACTOR AND ITS RECEPTOR

Granulocyte colony-stimulating factor (G-CSF) and its receptor (G-CSFR) control neutrophil production under basal circumstances and during episodes of bacterial

[a] Department of Hematology, Erasmus University Medical Center, Dr Molewaterplein 50 3015 GE, Rotterdam, The Netherlands; [b] Department of Tumor Immunology, Nijmegen Center for Molecular Life Sciences, Geert Grooteplein 28, 6525 GA, Nijmegen, The Netherlands
* Corresponding author. Department of Hematology, Erasmus University Medical Center, P.O. Box 1738, 3000 DR Rotterdam, The Netherlands.
E-mail address: i.touw@erasmusmc.nl

Hematol Oncol Clin N Am 27 (2013) 61–73
http://dx.doi.org/10.1016/j.hoc.2012.10.002
0889-8588/13/$ – see front matter © 2013 Elsevier Inc. All rights reserved.

hemonc.theclinics.com

infections, a condition referred to as "emergency" granulopoiesis.[1,2] Mice deficient for either G-CSF or G-CSFR suffer from severe neutropenia and are hyper-susceptible to infections, confirming the nonredundant role of the G-CSF/G-CSFR signaling axis in granulopoiesis and host defense.[3,4] G-CSFR is a single transmembrane protein and a member of the cytokine receptor superfamily.[5] The extracellular part contains an immunoglobulinlike (Ig-like) domain, a cytokine receptor homology domain (CRH domain) comprising a tryptophan serine repeat (WSXWS) and conserved cysteines, and 3 fibronectin type III (FNIII) modules (**Fig. 1**). G-CSF binds to G-CSFR in a 2:2 ratio, resulting in the homodimerization of receptor proteins required for G-CSFR activation.[6]

Like other members of this superfamily, G-CSFR activates the Janus kinase/signal transducer and activator of transcription (JAK/STAT), phosphoinositide-3 kinase/Akt (PI-3K/Akt) and p21^{RAS}/mitogen activated protein kinase (MAPK) signaling pathways.[7] In addition, a number of novel mechanisms involved in G-CSF signaling have been proposed.[8,9] The G-CSFR activates 3 members of the JAK family (JAK1, JAK2, and TYK2) and 2 STAT members (STAT3 and STAT5). The temporal kinetics of STAT3 and STAT5 activation are markedly distinct; whereas STAT3 stays activated on prolonged G-CSFR activation for hours (or even days), activation of STAT5 peaks after 15 minutes and then declines rapidly.[10] The gene encoding the suppressor of cytokine signaling 3 (SOCS3) is the most prominent direct transcriptional target of STAT3 in myeloid progenitors[11]; G-CSF–induced STAT5 targets in myeloid precursors remain ill-defined.

The cytoplasmic domain of the G-CSFR comprises 4 conserved tyrosine (Y) residues, which in the phosphorylated (p) state serve as binding sites for Src homology 2 (SH2) domain-containing signaling proteins.[12] These pY-coupled pathways are dispensable for G-CSF–induced granulopoiesis but orchestrate the signaling output of the G-CSFR, thereby controlling the proliferation/differentiation balance in neutrophil production under basal and emergency conditions.[13] For instance, pY729 (pY728 in mice) is a recruitment site for the inhibitory SOCS3 protein,[14] whereas the adapter proteins Shc and Grb2, involved in proliferation and prosurvival signaling through activation of p21Ras and PI-3K/Akt, bind to pY764 (pY763 in mice).[13,15,16] Details of pY-linked signaling pathways activated by the G-CSFR have been reviewed earlier[7,17] and are summarized in **Fig. 1**. Interestingly, SOCS3 does not only act in a classical negative feedback loop to attenuate G-CSF signaling, but is also involved in a transmodulatory role of the proinflammatory cytokine interferon-gamma (IFNγ) in the control of myelopoiesis.[18] While enhancing monocytic differentiation through activation of the transcription factors IRF8 and PU.1 in myeloid progenitor cells, IFNγ reduces G-CSF–driven neutrophil differentiation via STAT3-mediated induction of SOCS3.[18]

G-CSF RESPONSES AND G-CSFR DEFECTS IN SEVERE CONGENITAL NEUTROPENIA

Severe congenital neutropenia (SCN) is characterized by a promyelocytic maturation arrest in the bone marrow, leading to defective neutrophil production and life-threatening opportunistic bacterial infections. The underlying genetic defects causing this heterogeneous disease have been partly elucidated.[19,20] Mutations in the gene encoding neutrophil elastase (*ELANE*) are found in autosomal dominant and sporadic cases of SCN,[21] whereas mutations in the gene encoding HCLS1-associated protein X1 (*HAX1*) are responsible for the autosomal recessive form of SCN.[22] HAX1 is a mitochondrial protein and a prevailing hypothesis is that increased apoptosis of myeloid progenitor cells is the major underlying cellular principle responsible for the paucity of

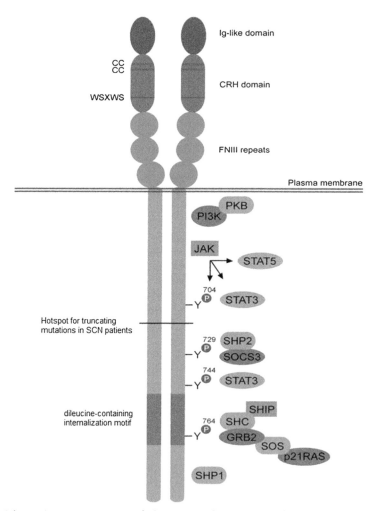

Fig. 1. Schematic representation of the activated G-CSFR. Modules in the extracellular domain characteristic of the cytokine receptor superfamily are shown (see main text). In the intracellular domain, the positioning of the tyrosine motifs and their connection to signaling pathways, the internalization domain, and the region affected by nonsense mutations in SCN are depicted.

mature neutrophils in HAX1-SCN.[22] How ELANE mutations fit into this hypothesis is not obvious. A number of possible explanations as to how mutant neutrophil elastase (NE) proteins cause neutropenia have been put forward. A current view is that mutant NE causes an unfolded protein response (UPR) in the endoplasmic reticulum (ER), leading to cell damage and apoptosis.[23] This hypothesis is supported by a recent study showing that mutant NE triggers the UPR in a transgenic mouse model and that inhibition of ERAD (ER-associated degradation) by the proteasome inhibitor bortezomib, allowing misfolded NE proteins to accumulate in cells, gave rise to reduced neutrophil levels.[24] Whether these experimental conditions bear significance for clinical SCN remains to be determined. G-CSF is used successfully in the clinic to alleviate neutropenia in patients with SCN, but there is a significant variation in dosage require-ments and efficacy.[25,26] Questions relevant for this review are how G-CSF therapy reverts the neutropenic phenotype and why G-CSF responses among patients are vari-able, even within the same genetic subtype of SCN.

A major clinical complication in SCN is the progression toward myelodysplastic syndrome (MDS) and acute myeloid leukemia (AML), emerging with the increased life expectancy owing to the reduced infection-related mortality.[23,24,27,28] In the 1990s, the first reports appeared in which nonsense mutations in the gene encoding the G-CSFR were described that result in the truncation of approximately 100 amino acids of the cytoplasmic domain of the receptor protein and that were associated with leukemic progression of the disease.[29–32] Studies in cell line and knock-in mouse models revealed that these truncated G-CSFRs were hampered in their ability to transduce signals controlling neutrophil differentiation in vitro and conferred hyperpro-liferative responses to G-CSF in vivo.[33–36] The mutations truncating the G-CSFR protein are acquired in hematopoietic clones during the neutropenic phase.[32] These clones may expand and give rise to leukemia, a process that will be further discussed later in this review. The truncation mutants are hampered in internalization and lack Y729-containing binding motif for SOCS3 (see **Fig. 1**). Activation of the G-CSFR trun-cation mutants results in drastically altered kinetics of STAT5 activation, that is, from transient (minutes) to sustained (hours) activation, and increased production of intra-cellular reactive oxygen species (ROS).[10,37] Importantly, STAT5 is essential for the clonal expansion of hematopoietic stem and progenitor cells in mice harboring the truncating G-CSFR-d715 mutation.[38] The elevated G-CSF–induced ROS levels in bone marrow cells expressing truncated G-CSFRs may potentially contribute to abnormal signaling by several mechanisms: by inactivation of oxidation sensitive phosphatases that negatively control growth factor signaling, by inducing responses to cellular stresses caused by ROS-induced damage, and by causing DNA damage leading to an elevated mutation rate in the HSC compartment. In the next paragraphs, these possibilities and their potential consequences for leukemic evolution of SCN are further discussed.

LYSOSOMAL ROUTING OF THE G-CSFR CONTROLLED BY RECEPTOR UBIQUITINATION

After activation of the G-CSFR at the plasma membrane, the G-CSF/G-CSFR complex is internalized. A conserved dileucine-containing stretch (STQPLL) at amino acid positions 749 to 754 within the G-CSFR cytoplasmic region is the major determinant responsible for clathrin-mediated receptor endocytosis.[39,40] The internalized G-CSF/ G-CSFR complex then enters the early endosome (or sorting endosome) compartment, where receptor complexes can undergo 2 fates: processing for lysosomal degradation or rerouting toward the plasma membrane.[41] Once present in early endosomes, the major portion of the G-CSF/G-CSFR complexes will be incorporated into so-called multivesicular bodies (MVBs). This process is governed by the endosomal sorting complex required for transport (ESCRT) machinery and involves ubiquitination on lysine (K) residues as a major protein modification, resulting in the interaction of the G-CSFR with multiple ubiquitin-binding adaptor proteins within the ESCRT complex.[41–44] A G-CSFR mutant lacking cytoplasmic lysine residues (mutant K5R) accumulates in early endosomes, emphasizing that lysine ubiquitination of the G-CSFR is crucial for routing toward late endosomes and lysosomes.[45] Additional mutational analysis showed that only the most membrane proximal lysine residue, K632, is critical for lyso-somal routing.[45,46] Ubiquitination is mediated by enzyme complexes consisting of ubiquitin-activating (E1), conjugating (E2), and ligating (E3) enzymes. The ring finger protein c-Cbl is the major E3 ligase involved in the ubiquitination of epidermal growth factor receptor (EGFR) and a number of other receptor tyrosine kinases.[47,48] c-Cbl has been implicated in the ubiquitination of some receptors of the cytokine receptor superfamily.[49–51] Alternative E3 ligase systems implicated in cytokine receptor ubiqui-tination include the Skp, Cullin, and F-box beta-Transducin repeat containing protein (beta-Trcp)[52] and receptor-associated ubiquitin ligase (RUL)[53]; however, neither of these E3-ligases has been implicated in lysosomal routing of the G-CSFR and, instead, a role for SOCS3 has been proposed.[45,46]

SOCS3 contains 2 distinct functional domains, the kinase inhibitory region (KIR), inhibiting JAK activity, and the SOCS box.[54–57] The SOCS box recruits the E3 ligase complex consisting of Elongin B/C, Cullin 5, and the RING finger protein Rbx2.[58] The SOCS3-SOCS box inhibits G-CSF responses in vitro and in vivo[59,60] and siRNA-mediated knockdown of SOCS3 expression reduces the ubiquitination of the membrane proximal lysine residue K632 of the G-CSFR. Furthermore, like mutant K632R, the G-CSFR mutant Y729F that is unable to bind SOCS3 was hampered in lysosomal routing.[45] Finally, the inhibitory effects of SOCS3 on G-CSF–induced STAT5 activation in reporter assays depended on the presence of G-CSFR-K632.[45,46] Taken together, these results suggest that SOCS3 controls lysosomal routing of G-CSFR by a mechanism involving the membrane proximal K632, a residue that is highly conserved in evolution and that is shared by multiple cytokine receptors.[46]

Protein ubiquitination is counteracted by de-ubiquitinating enzymes (DUBs). Expression of a family of DUBs comprising DUB1, DUB1A, DUB2, and DUB2A is controlled by cytokines.[61–64] G-CSF specifically induces the expression of DUB2A in myeloid cells, leading to de-ubiquitination and accumulation of the G-CSFR in early endosomes.[65] Based on these findings, a model has been proposed in which SOCS3 and DUB2A act in concert to control the dynamics of lysosomal routing of G-CSFR and signaling from the early endosome compartment.[65]

The G-CSFR truncation mutants, lacking both the STQPLL internalization motif and the tyrosine-based SOCS3 binding site (Y729), are severely hampered in internalization and lysosomal routing. In addition, they are more efficiently transported to the plasma membrane in the forward (biosynthetic) pathway.[39,66] Because of their prolonged half-life and residence time at the plasma membrane, it can be immediately inferred why the G-CSFR truncation mutants act dominantly over the wild-type form.[29] It remains a puzzle, however, why the G-CSFR mutations in SCN almost invariably affect forward and retrograde traffic of the G-CSFR. Strikingly, mutations in a number of neu-tropenia syndromes (eg, X-linked neutropenia [XLN], Hermansky-Pudlak syndrome type 2, Griscelli syndrome type 2, and p14 [ROBLD3] deficiency) all affect proteins involved in endosomal or lysosomal sorting.[20] Two patients with XLN treated with G-CSF have been reported who developed AML with G-CSFR mutations similar to those found in SCN.[67] Furthermore, HAX1 was initially identified as a protein interacting with HCLS1, a hematopoietic cell–specific cortactin-like protein that modulates endo-somal trafficking through its interaction with actin.[68] Taken together, these findings merit the hypothesis that abnormalities in endosomal and lysosomal sorting processes affect G-CSFR traffic and inhibit G-CSF responses in SCN and XLN and that G-CSF therapy favors the selection of G-CSFR mutant clones that escape this inhibition.

IMPACT OF INTRACELLULAR ROUTING ON G-CSFR FUNCTION

Apart from controlling the duration and amplitude of signals, intracellular trafficking of activated receptors has been shown to contribute to diversification of signaling by certain receptor systems.[41,42] Hence, an important question is how G-CSF signaling is dynamically controlled by intracellular trafficking and how this is affected in case of the internalization defective G-CSFR truncation mutants.

Local Control of G-CSF Signaling by Protein Tyrosine Phosphatase 1B

Two protein tyrosine phosphatases (PTPs) that are most frequently implicated in cytokine receptor signaling are the SH2-containing protein tyrosine phosphatase SHP1, encoded by *PTPN6*, and SHP2, encoded by *PTPN11*. Although SHP1 moderately inhibits G-CSFR signaling via a still unknown mechanism,[69] a role for SHP2's phosphatase activity has not been established. Rather, SHP2 promotes RAS/MAPK signaling by recruiting son of sevenless (SOS), a major nucleotide exchange factor for RAS, in a complex with GRB2 to the plasma membrane.[70] The RAS promoting activity of SHP2 is enhanced by mutations in *PTPN11* that cause Noonan syndrome and by *PTPN11* mutations acquired in patients with myeloproliferative disease or AML.[71] More recently, a prominent role for PTP1B in G-CSFR signaling has been discovered.[72] PTP1B has been originally implicated in metabolism and associated diseases, that is, obesity and diabetes and receptors inhibited by PTP1B include the insulin receptor (IR), platelet-derived growth factor receptor (PDGFR), insulin-like growth factor 1 receptor, and the EGFR.[73] In marked contrast to SHP1 and SHP2, PTP1B is not a cytoplasmic enzyme recruited to target proteins through pY-SH2 interactions, but is anchored to the outer membrane of the ER.[74] PTP1B robustly inhibits G-CSF–induced JAK/STAT activation, phosphorylation of G-CSFR tyrosines, and proliferation of myeloid progenitors in colony assays.[72] Confocal microscopy and in situ proximity ligation assays showed that exclusively the activated G-CSFRs in early endosomes, but not those at the plasma membrane, interacted with ER-resident PTP1B.[72] Inhibition of G-CSF responses by PTP1B thus depends on intracellular trafficking of the activated G-CSFR (**Fig. 2**).

Local Production of ROS and Effects on G-CSF Signaling

After G-CSF stimulation of myeloid progenitors, levels of ROS are rapidly elevated.[37] Apart from being crucial effectors in inflammatory responses, ROS are important regulators of signal transduction by affecting redox-sensitive enzyme activities, in particular protein tyrosine phosphatases. The NADPH oxidase (Nox) systems are major producers of H_2O_2, a main component of ROS.[75] Different Nox complexes (Nox1–5) have been identified that are localized in distinct subcellular compartments.[75] The Nox2 complex resides at the plasma membrane and is the source of H_2O_2 in oxidative burst formation in phagocytes. G-CSF activates this system via a mechanism involving phosphorylation and membrane translocation of p47^{phox}, a regulatory scaffold of the Nox2 complex.[37] The PI-3K/Akt pathway is responsible for phosphorylation of p47^{phox}. Activation of bone marrow cells expressing G-CSFR truncation mutants resulted in significantly higher ROS production compared with healthy controls.[37] Conceivably, the prolonged residence time at the plasma membrane as a result of defective internalization leading to sustained PI-3K/Akt activation will contribute to the elevated ROS production. In addition, the effects of ROS scavengers or antioxidant systems might be reduced as a result of the receptor truncations. Nox4 and Nox5 mainly reside at the ER.[76] The oxidation and inactivation of ER-resident PTP1B has been attributed to Nox4-mediated ROS production (see **Fig. 2**).[77,78]

Peroxiredoxins (Prdx) are antioxidant proteins that have been implicated in the control of signaling from receptor tyrosine kinases. Among the 6 mammalian Prdx proteins, Prdx1, 2, and 6 are cytosolic; Prdx3 is mitochondrial, and Prdx5 is peroxisomal.[79] Prdx2 physically interacts with PDGFR and attenuates negative regulation of PDGFR-mediated signaling.[80] Prdx1 has a similar effect and its activity is

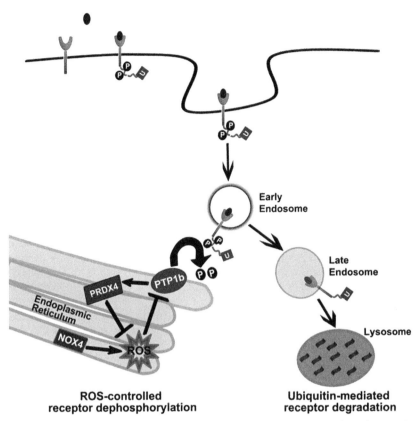

Fig. 2. Model of G-CSFR routing and involvement of PTP1B at the ER-early endosome interface. After ligand-induced activation and internalization, G-CSFRs enter the early endosome compartment, where they are subjected to 2 modulatory mechanisms: targeting to lysosomal degradation, a process depending on ubiquitination of the G-CSFR and its dephosphorylation by ER-resident PTP1B, the activity of which is controlled by locally produced ROS and the antioxidative activity of Prdx4.

inhibited by tyrosine phosphorylation through the PDGFR (and EGFR).[81] These observations have resulted in a model in which Prdx1 controls H_2O_2 levels and PTP activity in a spatially and temporally confined manner.[79]

Whether Prdx1 or Prdx2 exert similar roles in G-CSF signaling is unknown. Intriguingly, in a mammalian protein-protein interaction trap (MAPPIT) assay, Prdx4, but not Prdx1 or Prdx2, physically interacted with the most distal cytoplasmic region of G-CSFR.[72] Confocal imaging and in situ proximity ligation analysis showed that Prdx4 and G-CSFR colocalized after the activated G-CSFR routed to early endosomes. Prdx4 is predominantly, albeit not exclusively, localized in the ER.[82] Its antioxidant activity may therefore preferentially affect ER-resident proteins. A proposed function of Prdx4 is that it acts as a H_2O_2 sensor for protein folding in the ER.[79] Because the redox-sensitive PTP1B also is an ER-resident protein, and thus could be directly affected by local H_2O_2 levels, we asked whether Prdx4 might control the activity of PTP1B. G-CSF responses of Prdx4-deficient bone marrow cells were comparable to those of $Ptp1b^{-/-}$ bone marrow cells (ie, giving rise to significantly more and larger colonies in CFU-G assays).[72] Interestingly, PRDX4 expression is silenced by an epigenetic mechanism in human acute promyelocytic leukemia, suggesting that PRDX4 has a tumor suppressive role in the hematopoietic system.[83] It remains to be established whether PRDX4 affects the oxidation status of PTP1B and whether the interaction between PRDX4 and the G-CSFR C-terminus has physiologic relevance (eg, by tethering G-CSFRs), once present in early endosomes, to the ER. Irrespective of these unresolved issues, the ER clearly has an important regulatory function in G-CSF signaling, with the control of ROS levels as a major determinant of signal modulation at the ER-early endosome interface. The internalization-defective G-CSFR truncation mutants escape from this control mechanism in which PTP1B takes a central position.

G-CSFR MUTATIONS AND LEUKEMIC PROGRESSION OF SCN

The leukemia risk in SCN is alarming. The Severe Chronic Neutropenia International Registry (SCNIR) has monitored patients with SCN receiving G-CSF therapy since 1994.[24] In a study published in 2006, the cumulative incidence for MDS/AML after 10 years on G-CSF therapy was 21%.[27] Depending on the median dosage needed to reach an acceptable level of neutrophils, this group of patients was divided in poor G-CSF responders, with a 40% MDS/AML risk, and good G-CSF responders, with a lower (11%) risk of leukemic progression.[27] The G-CSFR mutation status was not reported in this study, but in an earlier long-term survey among 125 patients with SCN, G-CSFR mutations were reported in 34% of the patients in the neutropenic phase and in 18 (78%) of the 23 patients at the stage of MDS/AML.[84] The time between the first detection of the G-CSFR mutations and the diagnosis of MDS/AML varied considerably, and some patients harbored multiple G-CSFR mutations. The presence of multiple clones carrying distinct G-CSFR truncating mutations in patients with SCN patients is thought to be a risk factor for leukemic progression as well.

Whether regular monitoring of G-CSFR mutations to predict leukemic progression of SCN is clinically useful is still unresolved, but because patients with SCN/AML are refractory to therapy, it is essential to detect signs of malignant transformation before signs of leukemia become overt. In a recent study, serial hematopoietic samples of a patient with SCN who developed AML 17 years after initiation of G-CSF treatment were investigated by next-generation sequencing.[85] In the AML phase, 12 acquired nonsynonymous mutations were identified, 2 of which (in *LLGL2* and *ZC3H18*) co-occurred in a subpopulation of myeloid progenitor cells in the early SCN phase that already harbored a G-CSFR-d715 mutation. This population expanded in time, whereas other clones solely harboring distinct G-CSFR mutations (d717, d725, d730) disappeared from the bone marrow. Significantly, a new mutation (T595I) in the extracellular domain of G-CSFR on the already affected G-CSFR-d715 allele was present in the AML phase, which conferred growth factor independent proliferation to myeloid progenitors. These findings establish that progression from SCN toward AML is a multistep process with distinct mutations arising early during the SCN phase and others later in AML development. The sequential gain of the G-CSFR mutations (d715 and T595I) suggests that abnormal G-CSF signaling is a driver of leukemic transformation in this case of SCN.

SUMMARY

Although G-CSF has been routinely used for more than 2 decades to treat various types of SCN, the underlying mechanisms of G-CSF hyporesponsiveness or nonresponsiveness have remained largely elusive. A thorough understanding of the biology of G-CSFR activation and signaling function in relation to endosomal and lyso-somal trafficking will be useful to identify compounds that may act synergistically with G-CSF to overcome hyporesponsiveness or nonresponsiveness in SCN. Furthermore, it may shed light on how abnormal function of the G-CSFR, caused by mutations that prevent their normal intracellular trafficking, contribute to a premalignant state of hematopoietic stem and progenitor cells. Specifically, it remains to be resolved whether G-CSF merely drives the clonal expansion of the "sick" stem cells in SCN or actively contributes to the leukemic process through elevated production of ROS after activation of the truncated G-CSFR, leading to chronic DNA damage, acquisition of additional mutations, and rewiring of signaling and transcription regulatory processes.

REFERENCES

1. Demetri GD, Griffin JD. Granulocyte colony-stimulating factor and its receptor. Blood 1991;78(11):2791–808.
2. Lieschke GJ. CSF-deficient mice—what have they taught us? Ciba Found Symp 1997;204:60–74 [discussion: 7].
3. Lieschke GJ, Grail D, Hodgson G, et al. Mice lacking granulocyte colony-stimulating factor have chronic neutropenia, granulocyte and macrophage progenitor cell deficiency, and impaired neutrophil mobilization. Blood 1994; 84(6):1737–46.
4. Liu F, Wu HY, Wesselschmidt R, et al. Impaired production and increased apoptosis of neutrophils in granulocyte colony-stimulating factor receptor-deficient mice. Immunity 1996;5(5):491–501.
5. Bazan JF. Structural design and molecular evolution of a cytokine receptor super-family. Proc Natl Acad Sci U S A 1990;87(18):6934–8.
6. Layton JE, Hall NE. The interaction of G-CSF with its receptor. Front Biosci 2006; 11:3181–9.
7. Touw IP, van de Geijn GJ. Granulocyte colony-stimulating factor and its receptor in normal myeloid cell development, leukemia and related blood cell disorders. Front Biosci 2007;12:800–15.
8. Skokowa J, Cario G, Uenalan M, et al. LEF-1 is crucial for neutrophil granulocy-topoiesis and its expression is severely reduced in congenital neutropenia. Nat Med 2006;12(10):1191–7.
9. Skokowa J, Lan D, Thakur BK, et al. NAMPT is essential for the G-CSF-induced myeloid differentiation via a NAD(+)-sirtuin-1-dependent pathway. Nat Med 2009;15(2):151–8.
10. Hermans MH, Antonissen C, Ward AC, et al. Sustained receptor activation and hyperproliferation in response to granulocyte colony-stimulating factor (G-CSF) in mice with a severe congenital neutropenia/acute myeloid leukemia-derived mutation in the G-CSF receptor gene. J Exp Med 1999;189(4):683–92.
11. Lee CK, Raz R, Gimeno R, et al. STAT3 is a negative regulator of granulopoiesis but is not required for G-CSF-dependent differentiation. Immunity 2002;17(1): 63–72.
12. Ward AC, Smith L, de Koning JP, et al. Multiple signals mediate proliferation, differentiation, and survival from the granulocyte colony-stimulating factor receptor in myeloid 32D cells. J Biol Chem 1999;274(21):14956–62.
13. Hermans MH, van de Geijn GJ, Antonissen C, et al. Signaling mechanisms coupled to tyrosines in the granulocyte colony-stimulating factor receptor

orchestrate G-CSF-induced expansion of myeloid progenitor cells. Blood 2003; 101(7):2584–90.

14. Hortner M, Nielsch U, Mayr LM, et al. Suppressor of cytokine signaling-3 is recruited to the activated granulocyte-colony stimulating factor receptor and modulates its signal transduction. J Immunol 2002;169(3):1219–27.

15. de Koning JP, Schelen AM, Dong F, et al. Specific involvement of tyrosine 764 of human granulocyte colony-stimulating factor receptor in signal transduction mediated by p145/Shc/GRB2 or p90/GRB2 complexes. Blood 1996;87(1): 132–40.

16. de Koning JP, Soede-Bobok AA, Schelen AM, et al. Proliferation signaling and activation of Shc, p21Ras, and Myc via tyrosine 764 of human granulocyte colony-stimulating factor receptor. Blood 1998;91(6):1924–33.

17. Ward AC. The role of the granulocyte colony-stimulating factor receptor (G-CSF-R) in disease. Front Biosci 2007;12:608–18.

18. de Bruin AM, Libregts SF, Valkhof M, et al. IFNgamma induces monopoiesis and inhibits neutrophil development during inflammation. Blood 2012;119(6):1543–54.

19. Dale DC, Link DC. The many causes of severe congenital neutropenia. N Engl J Med 2009;360(1):3–5.

20. Klein C. Congenital neutropenia. Hematology Am Soc Hematol Educ Program 2009;344–50.

21. Horwitz MS, Duan Z, Korkmaz B, et al. Neutrophil elastase in cyclic and severe congenital neutropenia. Blood 2007;109(5):1817–24.

22. Klein C, Grudzien M, Appaswamy G, et al. HAX1 deficiency causes autosomal recessive severe congenital neutropenia (Kostmann disease). Nat Genet 2007; 39(1):86–92.

23. Freedman MH, Alter BP. Risk of myelodysplastic syndrome and acute myeloid leukemia in congenital neutropenias. Semin Hematol 2002;39(2):128–33.

24. Freedman MH, Bonilla MA, Fier C, et al. Myelodysplasia syndrome and acute myeloid leukemia in patients with congenital neutropenia receiving G-CSF therapy. Blood 2000;96(2):429–36.

25. Dale DC, Bonilla MA, Davis MW, et al. A randomized controlled phase III trial of recombinant human granulocyte colony-stimulating factor (filgrastim) for treatment of severe chronic neutropenia. Blood 1993;81(10):2496–502.

26. Dale DC, Cottle TE, Fier CJ, et al. Severe chronic neutropenia: treatment and follow-up of patients in the Severe Chronic Neutropenia International Registry. Am J Hematol 2003;72(2):82–93.

27. Rosenberg PS, Alter BP, Bolyard AA, et al. The incidence of leukemia and mortality from sepsis in patients with severe congenital neutropenia receiving long-term G-CSF therapy. Blood 2006;107(12):4628–35.

28. Zeidler C, Germeshausen M, Klein C, et al. Clinical implications of ELA2-, HAX1-, and G-CSF-receptor (CSF3R) mutations in severe congenital neutropenia. Br J Haematol 2009;144(4):459–67.

29. Dong F, Brynes RK, Tidow N, et al. Mutations in the gene for the granulocyte colony-stimulating–factor receptor in patients with acute myeloid leukemia preceded by severe congenital neutropenia. N Engl J Med 1995;333(8):487–93.

30. Dong F, Hoefsloot LH, Schelen AM, et al. Identification of a nonsense mutation in the granulocyte-colony-stimulating factor receptor in severe congenital neutropenia. Proc Natl Acad Sci U S A 1994;91(10):4480–4.

31. Dong F, Dale DC, Bonilla MA, et al. Mutations in the granulocyte colony-stimulating factor receptor gene in patients with severe congenital neutropenia. Leukemia 1997;11(1):120–5.

32. Tidow N, Pilz C, Teichmann B, et al. Clinical relevance of point mutations in the cytoplasmic domain of the granulocyte colony-stimulating factor receptor gene in patients with severe congenital neutropenia. Blood 1997;89(7):2369–75.
33. Dong F, van Buitenen C, Pouwels K, et al. Distinct cytoplasmic regions of the human granulocyte colony-stimulating factor receptor involved in induction of proliferation and maturation. Mol Cell Biol 1993;13(12):7774–81.
34. Fukunaga R, Ishizaka-Ikeda E, Nagata S. Growth and differentiation signals mediated by different regions in the cytoplasmic domain of granulocyte colony-stimulating factor receptor. Cell 1993;74(6):1079–87.
35. Hermans MH, Ward AC, Antonissen C, et al. Perturbed granulopoiesis in mice with a targeted mutation in the granulocyte colony-stimulating factor receptor gene associated with severe chronic neutropenia. Blood 1998;92(1):32–9.
36. McLemore ML, Poursine-Laurent J, Link DC. Increased granulocyte colony-stimulating factor responsiveness but normal resting granulopoiesis in mice carrying a targeted granulocyte colony-stimulating factor receptor mutation derived from a patient with severe congenital neutropenia. J Clin Invest 1998; 102(3):483–92.
37. Zhu QS, Xia L, Mills GB, et al. G-CSF induced reactive oxygen species involves Lyn-PI3-kinase-Akt and contributes to myeloid cell growth. Blood 2006;107(5): 1847–56.
38. Liu F, Kunter G, Krem MM, et al. Csf3r mutations in mice confer a strong clonal HSC advantage via activation of Stat5. J Clin Invest 2008;118(3):946–55.
39. Aarts LH, Roovers O, Ward AC, et al. Receptor activation and 2 distinct COOH-terminal motifs control G-CSF receptor distribution and internalization kinetics. Blood 2004;103(2):571–9.
40. Ward AC, van Aesch YM, Schelen AM, et al. Defective internalization and sustained activation of truncated granulocyte colony-stimulating factor receptor found in severe congenital neutropenia/acute myeloid leukemia. Blood 1999;93(2):447–58.
41. Sorkin A, von Zastrow M. Endocytosis and signalling: intertwining molecular networks. Nat Rev Mol Cell Biol 2009;10(9):609–22.
42. Polo S, Di Fiore PP. Endocytosis conducts the cell signaling orchestra. Cell 2006; 124(5):897–900.
43. Scita G, Di Fiore PP. The endocytic matrix. Nature 2010;463(7280):464–73.
44. Zwang Y, Yarden Y. Systems biology of growth factor-induced receptor endocytosis. Traffic 2009;10(4):349–63.
45. Irandoust MI, Aarts LH, Roovers O, et al. Suppressor of cytokine signaling 3 controls lysosomal routing of G-CSF receptor. EMBO J 2007;26(7):1782–93.
46. Wolfler A, Irandoust M, Meenhuis A, et al. Site-specific ubiquitination determines lysosomal sorting and signal attenuation of the granulocyte colony-stimulating factor receptor. Traffic 2009;10(8):1168–79.
47. Levkowitz G, Waterman H, Zamir E, et al. c-Cbl/Sli-1 regulates endocytic sorting and ubiquitination of the epidermal growth factor receptor. Genes Dev 1998; 12(23):3663–74.
48. Umebayashi K, Stenmark H, Yoshimori T. Ubc4/5 and c-Cbl continue to ubiquitinate EGF receptor after internalization to facilitate polyubiquitination and degradation. Mol Biol Cell 2008;19(8):3454–62.
49. Gesbert F, Malarde V, Dautry-Varsat A. Ubiquitination of the common cytokine receptor gammac and regulation of expression by an ubiquitination/deubiquitination machinery. Biochem Biophys Res Commun 2005;334(2):474–80.
50. Saur SJ, Sangkhae V, Geddis AE, et al. Ubiquitination and degradation of the thrombopoietin receptor c-Mpl. Blood 2010;115(6):1254–63.

51. Tanaka Y, Tanaka N, Saeki Y, et al. c-Cbl-dependent monoubiquitination and lyso-somal degradation of gp130. Mol Cell Biol 2008;28(15):4805–18.
52. Meyer L, Deau B, Forejtnikova H, et al. beta-Trcp mediates ubiquitination and degradation of the erythropoietin receptor and controls cell proliferation. Blood 2007;109(12):5215–22.
53. Friedman AD, Nimbalkar D, Quelle FW. Erythropoietin receptors associate with a ubiquitin ligase, p33RUL, and require its activity for erythropoietin-induced proliferation. J Biol Chem 2003;278(29):26851–61.
54. Fujimoto M, Naka T. Regulation of cytokine signaling by SOCS family molecules. Trends Immunol 2003;24(12):659–66.
55. Kile BT, Schulman BA, Alexander WS, et al. The SOCS box: a tale of destruction and degradation. Trends Biochem Sci 2002;27(5):235–41.
56. Sasaki A, Yasukawa H, Suzuki A, et al. Cytokine-inducible SH2 protein-3 (CIS3/SOCS3) inhibits Janus tyrosine kinase by binding through the N-terminal kinase inhibitory region as well as SH2 domain. Genes Cells 1999;4(6):339–51.
57. Yoshimura A, Naka T, Kubo M. SOCS proteins, cytokine signalling and immune regulation. Nat Rev Immunol 2007;7(6):454–65.
58. Kamura T, Maenaka K, Kotoshiba S, et al. VHL-box and SOCS-box domains determine binding specificity for Cul2-Rbx1 and Cul5-Rbx2 modules of ubiquitin ligases. Genes Dev 2004;18(24):3055–65.
59. Boyle K, Egan P, Rakar S, et al. The SOCS box of suppressor of cytokine signaling-3 contributes to the control of G-CSF responsiveness in vivo. Blood 2007;110(5):1466–74.
60. van de Geijn GJ, Gits J, Touw IP. Distinct activities of suppressor of cytokine signaling (SOCS) proteins and involvement of the SOCS box in controlling G-CSF signaling. J Leukoc Biol 2004;76(1):237–44.
61. Baek KH, Kim MS, Kim YS, et al. DUB-1A, a novel deubiquitinating enzyme subfamily member, is polyubiquitinated and cytokine-inducible in B-lymphocytes. J Biol Chem 2004;279(4):2368–76.
62. Baek KH, Mondoux MA, Jaster R, et al. DUB-2A, a new member of the DUB subfamily of hematopoietic deubiquitinating enzymes. Blood 2001;98(3):636–42.
63. Zhu Y, Lambert K, Corless C, et al. DUB-2 is a member of a novel family of cytokine-inducible deubiquitinating enzymes. J Biol Chem 1997;272(1):51–7.
64. Zhu Y, Pless M, Inhorn R, et al. The murine DUB-1 gene is specifically induced by the betac subunit of interleukin-3 receptor. Mol Cell Biol 1996;16(9):4808–17.
65. Meenhuis A, Verwijmeren C, Roovers O, et al. The deubiquitinating enzyme DUB2A enhances CSF3 signalling by attenuating lysosomal routing of the CSF3 receptor. Biochem J 2011;434(2):343–51.
66. Meenhuis A, Irandoust M, Wolfler A, et al. Janus kinases promote cell-surface expression and provoke autonomous signalling from routing-defective G-CSF receptors. Biochem J 2009;417(3):737–46.
67. Beel K, Vandenberghe P. G-CSF receptor (CSF3R) mutations in X-linked neutro-penia evolving to acute myeloid leukemia or myelodysplasia. Haematologica 2009;94(10):1449–52.
68. Uruno T, Zhang P, Liu J, et al. Haematopoietic lineage cell-specific protein 1 (HS1) promotes actin-related protein (Arp) 2/3 complex-mediated actin polymerization. Biochem J 2003;371(Pt 2):485–93.
69. Tapley P, Shevde NK, Schweitzer PA, et al. Increased G-CSF responsiveness of bone marrow cells from hematopoietic cell phosphatase deficient viable motheaten mice. Exp Hematol 1997;25(2):122–31.

70. Dance M, Montagner A, Salles JP, et al. The molecular functions of Shp2 in the Ras/Mitogen-activated protein kinase (ERK1/2) pathway. Cell Signal 2008;20(3): 453–9.
71. Neel BG, Gu H, Pao L. The 'Shp'ing news: SH2 domain-containing tyrosine phosphatases in cell signaling. Trends Biochem Sci 2003;28(6):284–93.
72. Palande K, Roovers O, Gits J, et al. Peroxiredoxin-controlled G-CSF signalling at the endoplasmic reticulum-early endosome interface. J Cell Sci 2011;124(Pt 21): 3695–705.
73. Stuible M, Tremblay ML. In control at the ER: PTP1B and the down-regulation of RTKs by dephosphorylation and endocytosis. Trends Cell Biol 2010;20:672–9.
74. Frangioni JV, Beahm PH, Shifrin V, et al. The nontransmembrane tyrosine phosphatase PTP-1B localizes to the endoplasmic reticulum via its 35 amino acid C-terminal sequence. Cell 1992;68(3):545–60.
75. Bedard K, Krause KH. The NOX family of ROS-generating NADPH oxidases: physiology and pathophysiology. Physiol Rev 2007;87(1):245–313.
76. Chen K, Kirber MT, Xiao H, et al. Regulation of ROS signal transduction by NADPH oxidase 4 localization. J Cell Biol 2008;181(7):1129–39.
77. Mahadev K, Zilbering A, Zhu L, et al. Insulin-stimulated hydrogen peroxide reversibly inhibits protein-tyrosine phosphatase 1b in vivo and enhances the early insulin action cascade. J Biol Chem 2001;276(4):21938–42.
78. Meng TC, Buckley DA, Galic S, et al. Regulation of insulin signaling through reversible oxidation of the protein-tyrosine phosphatases TC45 and PTP1B. J Biol Chem 2004;279(36):37716–25.
79. Rhee SG, Woo HA, Kil IS, et al. Peroxiredoxin functions as a peroxidase and a regulator and sensor of local peroxides. J Biol Chem 2012;287(7):4403–10.
80. Choi MH, Lee IK, Kim GW, et al. Regulation of PDGF signalling and vascular remodelling by peroxiredoxin II. Nature 2005;435(7040):347–53.
81. Woo HA, Yim SH, Shin DH, et al. Inactivation of peroxiredoxin I by phosphorylation allows localized H(2)O(2) accumulation for cell signaling. Cell 2010;140(4): 517–28.
82. Tavender TJ, Sheppard AM, Bulleid NJ. Peroxiredoxin IV is an endoplasmic reticulum-localized enzyme forming oligomeric complexes in human cells. Biochem J 2008;411(1):191–9.
83. Palande KK, Beekman R, van der Meeren LE, et al. The antioxidant protein peroxiredoxin 4 is epigenetically down regulated in acute promyelocytic leukemia. PLoS One 2011;6(1):e16340.
84. Germeshausen M, Ballmaier M, Welte K. Incidence of CSF3R mutations in severe congenital neutropenia and relevance for leukemogenesis: results of a long-term survey. Blood 2007;109(1):93–9.
85. Beekman R, Valkhof MG, Sanders MA, et al. Sequential gain of mutations in severe congenital neutropenia progressing to acute myeloid leukemia. Blood 2012;119(22):5071–7.

Defective G-CSFR Signaling Pathways in Congenital Neutropenia

Julia Skokowa, MD, PhD*, Karl Welte, MD

KEYWORDS

- Severe congenital neutropenia • G-CSFR signaling • LEF-1 • HCLS1 (HS1)
- NAMPT-SIRT1 • ELANE • STAT5

KEY POINTS

- Severely reduced expression of myeloid-specific transcription factors, lymphoid enhancer binding factor 1 (LEF-1) and C/EBPα.
- Severely reduced expression and functions of HCLS1 protein.
- Severely reduced expression of neutrophil elastase (NE) protein.
- Dramatic compensatory up-regulation of the nicotinamide phosphoribosyltransferase (NAMPT)/NAD⁺/SIRT pathway, leading to continuous activation of emergency granulopoiesis via the transcription factor C/EBPβ.
- Hyperactivation of STAT5 protein by tyrosine phosphorylation.

GRANULOCYTE COLONY-STIMULATING FACTOR RECEPTOR SIGNALING IS SEVERELY AFFECTED IN CONGENITAL NEUTROPENIA PATIENTS

Granulocyte colony-stimulating factor (G-CSF) receptor (G-CSFR) activation with ligand binding induces myeloid cell proliferation, survival, and differentiation.[1] Acquired somatic mutations within the CSF3R gene and/or defects in the CSF3R downstream signaling pathways abrogate myeloid differentiation and might lead to either leukemic transformation or congenital neutropenia (CN).[2,3] In CN patients, the levels of G-CSF mRNA in mononuclear cells, the concentrations of biologically active G-CSF in serum, and the CSF3R expression in myeloid cells are considerably elevated compared with healthy individuals.[4,5] Daily injections of pharmacologic doses of G-CSF (100–1000 times higher than physiologic levels), however, are needed to increase peripheral blood neutrophil counts to greater than 1000/µL in CN patients.[3] Therefore, the authors assume that G-CSFR downstream signaling is severely defective in CN, leading to maturation arrest of granulopoiesis.

Disclosure: We have nothing to disclose.
Department of Molecular Hematopoiesis, Children's Hospital, Hannover Medical School, Carl-Neuberg Strasse 1, Hannover 30625, Germany
* Corresponding author.
E-mail address: skokowa.julia@mh-hannover.de

COMMON PATHOMECHANISM OF DEFECTIVE GRANULOPOIESIS IN CONGENITAL NEUTROPENIA PATIENTS HARBORING EITHER ELANE OR HAX1 MUTATIONS

Autosomal dominant mutations in the *ELANE* and autosomal recessive mutations in the *HAX1* have been identified in a majority of CN patients (60% and 10%, respectively).[6,7] Mutations in other genes, such as *G6PC3, GPT1, TAZ1, WAS,* and so forth, are rare and are discussed in articles elsewhere in this issue by Boztug and colleagues. This article predominantly reports on data from patients harboring *ELANE* and *HAX1* mutations. Ultimate defects in intracellular signaling pathways downstream of either *ELANE* or *HAX1* mutations leading to the defective granulopoiesis were elusive until recently. Clinical observations revealed that CN patients harboring either *ELANE* or *HAX1* mutations have comparable bone marrow (BM) morphology, responses to G-CSF therapy, and requirements of G-CSF dosages.[3] Also the risk (approximately 20%) of developing leukemias is comparable in both patient subgroups. Based on these clinical data, the authors suggest a common pathomechanism of defective G-CSF–triggered granulopoiesis downstream of both mutated genes (**Fig. 1**). In the past few years, the authors identified several novel signaling pathways that are activated by G-CSF in healthy individuals and are dramatically deregulated in hematopoietic cells of CN patients, leading to ineffective granulopoiesis.

A LACK OF LEF-1 AND C/EBPα TRANSCRIPTION FACTOR EXPRESSION IN MYELOID CELLS OF CONGENITAL NEUTROPENIA PATIENTS

The authors aimed to identifying signaling pathways or related myeloid transcription factors that are severely reduced in CN patients causing abnormal granulopoiesis downstream of the *ELANE* or *HAX1* mutations. mRNA expression profiles were compared between CD33$^+$ BM myeloid cells (predominantly promyelocytes) of CN patients, healthy individuals, and patients with neutropenia other than CN (cyclic neutropenia, idiopathic neutropenia, or neutropenia due to metabolic defects, such as glycogenosis type Ib); all groups were treated or not with G-CSF. Severely diminished expression and functions of the transcription factors, LEF-1 and C/EBPα, in myeloid cells of CN patients were identified compared with all other studied groups.[8] LEF-1

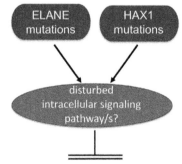

"maturation arrest" of granulocytic precursors
leading to congenital neutropenia

Fig. 1. Common pathomechanism of defective granulopoiesis in CN patients harboring either *ELANE* or *HAX1* mutations. CN patients harboring either *ELANE* or *HAX1* mutations have similar BM and clinical phenotype. Therefore, the authors suggest a common pathomechanism of defective G-CSF–triggered granulopoiesis (common defective intracellular signaling pathways) downstream of both mutated genes.

expression was abrogated in CN patients harboring either *ELANE* or *HAX1* mutations, which suggested LEF-1 as a possible common candidate factor for defective G-CSF signaling in both groups of CN patients. The authors demonstrated markedly diminished G-CSF–triggered in vitro granulocytic differentiation of CD34$^+$ cells of healthy individuals after knockdown of LEF-1. At the same time, LEF-1 rescue in hematopoietic cells of CN patients restored maturation arrest of granulopoiesis.[8] Furthermore, LEF-1 was found to regulate granulopoiesis by direct binding to the gene promoter of the known granulocyte-specific transcription factor C/EBPα[9] and activated expression of C/EBPα in myeloid cells (**Fig. 2**). In CN patients, C/EBPα expression was also severely diminished, representing a possible reason for the defective granulocytic differentiation.

IMBALANCE IN THE TRANSCRIPTIONAL REGULATION OF GRANULOPOIETIC VERSUS MONOPOIETIC DIFFERENTIATION PROGRAMS OF MYELOID PROGENITOR CELLS OF CONGENITAL NEUTROPENIA PATIENTS

CN patients have elevated levels of peripheral blood monocytes, which can be explained by compensatory monocytosis due to diminished neutrophil counts and functions.[10] Another reason for elevated production of monocytes and diminished granulopoiesis is deregulated expression of lineage-specific (granulocyte-specific and monocyte-specific) transcription factors in myeloid progenitor cells of CN patients. Proper regulation of granulopoiesis versus monopoiesis is tightly regulated by balanced expression of granulocyte-specific transcription factors (eg, C/EBPα) and monocyte-specific transcription factors (eg, PU.1).[11–13] Thus, C/EBPα expression levels elevated above PU.1 levels lead to granulocytic differentiation, but prevalence of PU.1 expression above C/EBPα levels shifts differentiation toward monocytes. The authors found elevated levels of PU.1 expression and severe diminished levels of C/EBPα in myeloid progenitor cells of CN patients, which may be a reason for elevated monocyte production and defective granulopoiesis in these patients. Previously, it has been demonstrated that LEF-1 binds to the upstream regulatory element

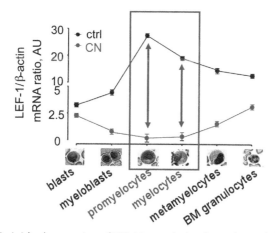

Fig. 2. Severely diminished expression of LEF-1 transcription factor in myeloid cells of patients with severe CN. BM cells in different stages of myeloid differentiation were isolated from BM smears using laser-assisted single-cell picking, and LEF-1 levels were analyzed by quantitative reverse transcriptase–polymerase chain reaction. AU, arbitrary units; ctrl, healthy controls (n = 10); CN, CN patients (n = 12).

of the *PU.1* gene promoter, inhibiting PU.1 expression.[14] Thus, a lack of LEF-1 in myeloid cells of CN patients could cause up-regulation of PU.1 and down-regulation of C/EBPα expression, inducing a shift from granulocytopoiesis toward monocytopoiesis of myeloid progenitors in CN patients.

The authors and other investigators also demonstrated dose-dependent effects of LEF-1 in G-CSFR–triggered myelopoiesis: defective LEF-1 expression causes neutropenia, but overexpression of LEF-1 results in elevated proliferation of human hematopoietic cells and development of acute myeloid leukemia (AML) in a mouse model.[8,15] Inhibition of LEF-1 by small hairpin RNA (shRNA) induces apoptosis and cell cycle arrest of the AML cell lines and primary AML blasts. LEF-1 belongs to the LEF-1/T-cell factor (TCF) family (TCF-1, TCF-3, and TCF-4) of high mobility group (HMG) domain transcription factors of the Wnt signaling pathway that recognize DNA consensus motifs through HMG box DNA-binding domain. LEF-1 does not have a transactivation domain but contains a DNA-binding domain.[16–24] Therefore, it requires additional interaction partners with a transactivation domain to activate target genes. The best-known interaction partner of LEF-1 is β-catenin. The authors demonstrated, however, that activation of C/EBPα and subsequent stimulation of granulopoiesis by LEF-1 are β-catenin independent. LEF-1 lacking β-catenin binding domain was able to activate C/EBPα.[8]

HCLS1, THE HEMATOPOIETIC-SPECIFIC INTERACTION PARTNER OF LEF-1, CONNECTS *HAX1* MUTATIONS WITH DIMINISHED LEF-1 EXPRESSION

The authors were interested in identifying hematopoiesis-specific interaction partners of LEF-1. Moreover, it was unclear why mutations in the ubiquitously expressed protein HAX1 induce isolated neutropenia and no defects in other tissues. The mechanism downstream of *HAX1* mutations leading to defective LEF-1 expression was also unknown. The authors performed screening of candidate proteins with hematopoiesis-specific expression and activity, which can interact and regulate LEF-1 transcription factor, and found that hematopoietic cell-specific Lyn substrate 1 (HCLS1 or HS1)[25] interacted with LEF-1 protein, transporting LEF-1 into the nucleus with G-CSF stimulation and subsequently inducing LEF-1 autoregulation, C/EBPα activation, and granulocytic differentiation.[26] HCLS1 protein is expressed at high levels in human myeloid cells, is associated with Lyn and Syk, and is phosphorylated on stimulation with G-CSF. HAX1 is a HCLS1-associated protein X1[27] and, in CN patients with *HAX1* mutations, the authors found profound defects in the G-CSF–triggered phosphorylation of HCLS1, which subsequently leads to abrogated nuclear transport of LEF-1, reduced autoregulation of LEF-1, and neutropenia.[26] Therefore, the authors were able to identify a direct link between *HAX1* mutations, defective LEF-1 expression, and isolated neutropenia in CN patients. Moreover, the authors identified one hematopoietic-specific interaction partner of LEF-1.[26]

What are the main functions of HCLS1? HCLS1 belongs to the SRC homology 3 domain adapter proteins and can initiate activation of receptor-coupled tyrosine kinases.[28,29] The proline-rich region is the site of tyrosine phosphorylation of HCLS1 and, therefore, responsible for many interactions with SH2-domain–containing proteins.[28,29] The phosphorylation sites have been implicated in the regulation of the HCLS1 activity through the connection with diverse tyrosine kinases, such as Syk, Lyn, and Lck, and the adapter proteins, such as Grb2.[28–34] Phosphorylation of HCLS1 on Tyr-397 by Syk and Lyn leads to HCLS1 translocation into the nucleus.[35] Helix-turn-helix repeat and coiled-coil domains of HCLS1 are required for binding to

F-actin and activation of the Arp2/3 complex.[25,28,29,36] HCLS1 protein is also associated with PI3K/Akt pathway. Knowing the functions of the HCLS1 protein, the authors further analyzed if HCLS1 is involved in the G-CSF–triggered F-actin rearrangement. Previously, the authors demonstrated that F-actin assembly induced by G-CSF treatment is severely impaired in myeloid cells of CN patients.[37] G-CSF treatment of CD34$^+$ cells of healthy individuals led to a rapid and transient increase in F-actin content. As seen in CN patients, basal F-actin levels were significantly increased in CD34$^+$ cells after knockdown of HAX1 or HCLS1. G-CSF was unable, however, to regulate the amount of F-actin in the absence of HAX1 or HCLS1. Therefore, the authors concluded that HCLS1 and HAX1 are important for G-CSF-induced F-actin assembly and that, in CN patients, mutations in the *HAX1* with subsequent defects in HCLS1 activation may contribute to abnormal F-actin.

Because HCLS1 is also associated with PI3K/Akt pathway[38] and PI3K/Akt is activated by G-CSF,[39] the authors further analyzed if HCLS1 is involved in G-CSF–triggered activation of PI3K/Akt signaling and found that treatment of CD34$^+$ cells with G-CSF led to phosphorylation of PI3K p85 (on Tyr458) and of Akt (on Ser473), which were both markedly reduced in cells transduced with HCLS1-specific or HAX1-specific shRNA. Similarly, much lower amounts of G-CSF–dependent phospho-PI3K p85 (Tyr458) and phospho-Akt (Ser473) were detected in CD34$^+$ cells of patients with CN compared with cells from healthy individuals. Thus, the authors identified a new essential player in the G-CSFR signaling pathway that is involved in nuclear transport and activation of LEF-1 transcription factor, activation of PI3K/Akt pathway, and deregulation of F-actin assembly. Similar to LEF-1, the functions of HCLS1 are dose dependent (**Fig. 3**). Thus, the authors also detected dramatically elevated HCLS1 protein levels in blasts of AML patients. A large cohort of AML patients also has insertion in the HCLS1 gene, which is localized in the proline-rich region of the

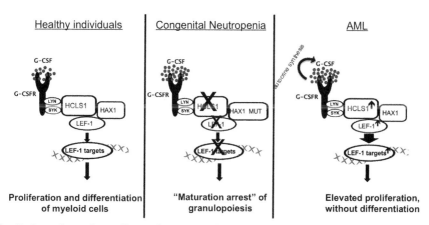

Fig. 3. Dose-dependent effects of HCLS1 and LEF-1 in myelopoiesis. HCLS1 interacts with HAX1 and LEF-1 proteins and on stimulation with G-CSF is tyrosine phosphorylated and transports LEF-1 into the nucleus, inducing LEF-1 autoregulation and proper proliferation and differentiation of myeloid cells (*left*). In patients with CN expression, functions of HCLS1 are severely diminished due to the mutations in the *HAX1* gene. HCLS1 and HAX1 are not able to bind LEF-1. Therefore, nuclear transport and autoregulation of LEF-1 are defective, leading to a maturation arrest of granulopoiesis (*middle*). In AML patients, HCLS1 is hyperactivated because of autocrine production of cytokines by AML blast or activating insertion in exon 12 of the HCLS1 gene. This leads to hyperproliferation of malignant cells (*right*).

HCLS1 protein. This insertion has been described as transmitting an accelerated B-cell receptor signaling in B lymphocytes inducing receptor-independent activation.[40] Similar hyperactivating events may be responsible for hyperproliferation of AML blasts.

NICOTINAMIDE PHOSPHORIBOSYLTRANSFERASE–DEPENDENT COMPENSATORY HYPERACTIVATION OF EMERGENCY GRANULOPOIESIS IN CONGENITAL NEUTROPENIA PATIENTS

The authors were further interested in how G-CSF treatment can overcome maturation arrest of granulopoiesis in CN patients despite the absence of LEF-1 and C/EBPα in myeloid cells. The hypothesis was that for responses to physiologic dosages of G-CSF, additional compensatory mechanisms, which are independent of LEF-1 and C/EBPα, should be activated with G-CSF treatment in CN patients. In the search for such mechanisms, the authors identified NAMPT[41–43] as an essential enzyme mediating G-CSF–triggered granulopoiesis in healthy individuals and in CN patients.[44] Treatment of healthy individuals with G-CSF resulted in up-regulation of NAMPT levels in myeloid cells via STAT3 and subsequent release of NAMPT into the plasma. At the same time, intracellular NAMPT and NAD$^+$ amounts in myeloid cells, as well as plasma NAMPT and NAD$^+$ levels, were even more dramatically elevated by G-CSF treatment of individuals with CN. The molecular events triggered by NAMPT included elevation of NAD$^+$, NAD$^+$-dependent activation of protein deacetylase sirtuin-1 (SIRT1), binding of SIRT1 to the myeloid-specific transcription factors, C/EBPα and C/EBPβ, and subsequent activation of these transcription factors (**Fig. 4**). G-CSF and G-CSFR are target genes of C/EBPs and treatment of myeloid cells with NAMPT induced autocrine C/EBP-triggered production of G-CSF and expression of G-CSFR, providing a feedback loop of G-CSF:G-CSFR signaling. C/EBPα transcription factor regulates steady-state granulopoiesis and, in cases of bacterial infections or situations that require rapid granulocyte production, emergency granulopoiesis triggered by C/EBPβ is activated.[45] In patients with CN, expression of C/EBPα transcription factor is severely diminished due to a lack of LEF-1[8]; therefore steady-state granulopoiesis could not be activated. G-CSF treatment, however, induces expression of C/EBPβ transcription factor in these patients via NAMPT and SIRT1 and operates via emergency arm of granulopoietic signaling. Because, for emergency granulopoiesis, continuous presence of the strong activation stimulus is required, G-CSF should be administered daily in high therapeutic doses to reach sufficient granulocyte numbers in CN patients (**Fig. 5**). Thus, another novel player in G-CSF signal transduction pathway has been identified and an important

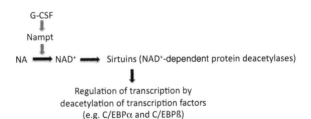

Fig. 4. Effects of NAMPT and G-CSF on the posttranslational protein modification via deacetylation. G-CSF induces NAMPT synthesis by induction of STAT3 binding to the NAMPT gene promoter. NAMPT converts nicotinamide (NA) into NAD$^+$. NAD$^+$ activates NAD$^+$-dependent protein deacetylases sirtuins. Sirtuins can bind and activate transcription factors by deacetylation and thus regulate gene transcription.

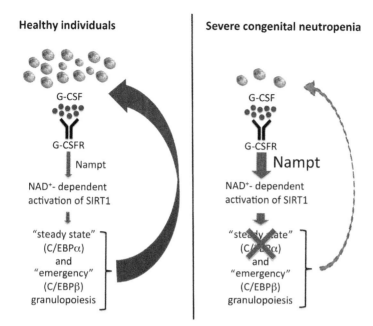

Healthy individuals

Severe congenital neutropenia

Fig. 5. Compensatory activation of the emergency granulopoiesis in CN patients by NAMPT. In healthy individuals, treatment with G-CSF triggers synthesis of Nampt, subsequent elevation of NAD⁺ levels, activation of SIRT1, binding of SIRT1 to the myeloid-specific transcription factors C/EBPα (responsible for the steady-state granulopoiesis) and C/EBPβ (main inducer of emergency granulopoiesis), and activation of these transcription factors. G-CSF and G-CSFR are target genes of C/EBPs, and treatment of myeloid cells with NAMPT induced autocrine C/EBP-triggered production of G-CSF and expression of G-CSFR, providing a feedback loop of G-CSF:G-CSFR signaling (*left*). In CN patients, expression of C/EBPα transcription factor is severely diminished due to a lack of LEF-1; therefore steady-state granulopoiesis could not be activated. G-CSF treatment, however, induces expression of C/EBPβ transcription factor in these patients via NAMPT and SIRT1 and operating via emergency arm of granulopoietic signaling, which is not as potent as steady state (*right*).

role of deacetylation of myeloid-specific transcription factors in G-CSFR–triggered myeloid differentiation has been established. Modulation of protein deacetylation by treatment of neutropenia patients with nicotinamide (vitamin B_3), which is converted into NAD⁺ by the enzyme NAMPT, could be applied.

THE ROLE OF THE *ELANE* MUTATIONS IN THE PATHOGENESIS OF CONGENITAL NEUTROPENIA

The *ELANE* encodes protein NE, which is a serine protease secreted by neutrophils. Although autosomal dominant mutations in the *ELANE* in patients with CN were initially described in 1999, the definitive pathomechanism downstream of these mutations leading to neutropenia is still unclear. To date, more than 60 different mutations have been identified in the *ELANE*. It is unclear why the same *ELANE* mutations have been found in two different hematopoietic syndromes, CN and cyclic neutropenia. There are several critical arguments concerning the role of the *ELANE* mutations in the pathogenesis of CN: (1) there is no clear genotype-phenotype correlation, and different *ELANE* mutations confer widely disparate effects on NE enzymatic activity; (2) analysis of mutated recombinant NE proteins has shown no evident changes in protein stability or substrate specificity and no consistent effects on glycosylation, and proteolytic activity retains some mutants compared with the wild-type protein; and (3) gene targeting of *ELANE* has failed to reproduce neutropenic phenotype in mice.[46–49] Nevertheless, some studies have proposed that mutant *ELANE* triggers accelerate apoptosis of granulocyte precursors or lead to cytoplasmatic accumulation of the altered protein, disturbance of intracellular trafficking, activation of the unfolded protein response (UPR), and induction of endoplasmic reticulum (ER) stress-triggered apoptosis.[50–52]

Recently, the authors reported severely diminished levels of the ELANE mRNA expression in myeloid cells as well as of the NE protein in plasma of CN patients harboring *ELANE* or *HAX1* mutations.[53] *ELANE* and NE levels in patients with CyN, however, in which *ELANE* is mutated in most patients, were comparable with the levels in healthy persons. Therefore, diminished levels of NE may be responsible in part for the defective granulopoiesis in CN. NE is a protease stored in primary granules of neutrophilic granulocytes that are formed during the promyelocytic phase of granulocyte differentiation.[54] NE is released after neutrophil activation and can cleave multiple substrates, including cytokines and chemokines (G-CSF and SDF-1α)[55–57] as well as cell-surface proteins (G-CSFR, VCAM, c-kit, and CXCR4).[56–60] G-CSF administration induces an increase in the level of NE in BM myeloid cells and the subsequent mobilization of BM stem cells to the peripheral blood. By cleavage of the chemokine receptor CXCR4 and its ligand, SDF-1α, NE negatively regulates SDF-1α/CXCR4 signaling, which plays a crucial role in the retention of hematopoietic cells within the BM and their mobilization to the peripheral blood.[61–64] The degree of mobilization positively correlates with the down-regulation of the surface expression of CXCR4 by mobilized cells. G-CSF–triggered stem cell mobilization (as a backup treatment before allogenic BM transplantation) is diminished in CN patients, despite a temporary 10-fold increase in the daily administered G-CSF dose (K.W., unpublished data, December 2000). The authors found elevated surface expression of CXCR4 on CD34$^+$ cells of CN patients that was normalized by incubation of cells with recombinant human NE. Therefore, abrogated stem cell mobilization on G-CSF treatment may be due to defective NE synthesis followed by elevated expression of CXCR4 on the hematopoietic stem cells in CN patients.

THE ROLE OF THE DISTURBED G-CSFR SIGNALING IN THE LEUKEMOGENIC TRANSFORMATION IN CONGENITAL NEUTROPENIA PATIENTS

CN is also considered a preleukemic syndrome, because CN patients are at increased risk of developing AML (cumulative incidence, approximately 20%).[65] Whether and how G-CSF affects this predisposition remain unclear. The authors found a significant and sustained elevation in the levels of phospho-STAT5 in hematopoietic CD34$^+$ cells of CN patients harboring *HAX1* or *ELA2* mutations compared with those of healthy individuals (Gupta and colleagues, unpublished data, ASH Meeting 2010). Phospho-STAT5 levels were even higher in a CN patient who subsequently developed AML. CN patients require pharmacologically high doses of G-CSF for treatment, because steady-state granulopoiesis via C/EBPα is defective in these patients.[8] High doses of G-CSF are required to support emergency granulopoiesis via C/EBPβ, which is not affected in CN.[44] High levels of G-CSF act as a persistent trigger for activation of JAK kinases associated with G-CSFR signaling, and these hyperactivated JAK kinases can lead to elevated levels of phospho-STAT5 in CN cells. The authors demonstrated that G-CSF treatment induces significantly higher and sustained levels of phospho-STAT5 in CD34$^+$ cells of CN patients compared with healthy individuals

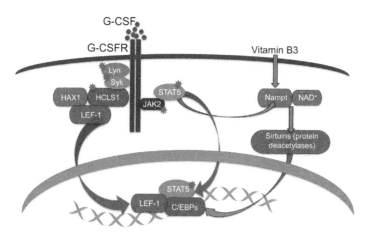

Fig. 6. New G-CSFR signaling pathways in myelopoiesis. LEF-1 transcription factor is essential for G-CSFR–triggered granulocytic differentiation by activation of C/EBPα expression. HCLS1 and HAX1 proteins interact with LEF-1 protein transporting LEF-1 into the nucleus, where LEF-1 binds to its own promoter and promoters of LEF-1 target genes. G-CSF also activates another signaling pathway through STAT3-dependent induction of NAMPT, NAD$^+$, and sirtuins. By this, G-CSF stimulates deacetylation of myeloid transcription factors. Hyperactivation of STAT5 proteins by continuous treatment of cells with G-CSF may induce leukemogenic intracellular events.

and also found diminished expression of SOCS3, which is normally terminates STAT5 phosporylation, in CN myeloid cells; previously the authors demonstrated elevated levels of JAK2 in CN neutrophils.[66] These events may contribute to elevated phosphorylation of STAT5 in CN. Additionally, ELA2 mutations in myeloid cells of CN patients lead to cytoplasmic accumulation of a nonfunctional elastase protein and disturbance of intracellular trafficking, followed by activation of the UPR and ER stress.[50–52] ER stress/UPR are also associated with induction of the JAK2/STAT5 signaling pathway.[67] Therefore, UPR might also induce sustained hyperphosphorylation of STAT5 in CN patients.

Consistent with hyperactivated STAT5 having been implicated in various hematological malignancies, including AML, and in myeloproliferative disorders,[68] the authors' data demonstrating that even higher levels of phospho-STAT5 in CN/AML patients than in CN patients without AML might indicate that leukemic transformations secondary to CN are, in part, a consequence of elevated activation of STAT5.

The other possible reason for leukemogenic transformation is elevated NAMPT levels with subsequent hyperactivation of protein deacetylases (described previously). The effects of NAMPT are strictly dose dependent. The authors and other investigators previously described NAMPT/SIRT1,2-dependent deacetylation of tumor suppressor protein p53,[69] proto-oncogene FOXO3a,[70] and Akt[71] proteins. These events may contribute to the leukemogenesis in CN patients.

SUMMARY

Several signaling systems have been identified that are defective or hyperactivated in myeloid cells of patients with CN (**Fig. 6**):

1. Severely reduced expression of myeloid-specific transcription factors LEF-1 and C/EBPα
2. Severely reduced expression and functions of HCLS1 protein

3. Severely reduced expression of NE protein
4. Dramatic compensatory up-regulation of the NAMPT/NAD$^+$/SIRT pathway leading to continuous activation of emergency granulopoiesis via the transcription factor C/EBPβ
5. Hyperactivation of STAT5 protein by tyrosine phosphorylation.

REFERENCES

1. Welte K, Gabrilove J, Bronchud MH, et al. Filgrastim (r-metHuG-CSF): the first 10 years. Blood 1996;88:1907–29.
2. Dong F, Brynes RK, Tidow N, et al. Mutations in the gene for the granulocyte colony-stimulating-factor receptor in patients with acute myeloid leukemia preceded by severe congenital neutropenia. N Engl J Med 1995;333:487–93.
3. Welte K, Zeidler C, Dale DC. Severe congenital neutropenia. Semin Hematol 2006;43:189–95.
4. Mempel K, Pietsch T, Menzel T, et al. Increased serum levels of granulocyte colony-stimulating factor in patients with severe congenital neutropenia. Blood 1991;77:1919–22.
5. Kyas U, Pietsch T, Welte K. Expression of receptors for granulocyte colony-stimulating factor on neutrophils from patients with severe congenital neutropenia and cyclic neutropenia. Blood 1992;79:1144–7.
6. Dale DC, Person RE, Bolyard AA, et al. Mutations in the gene encoding neutrophil elastase in congenital and cyclic neutropenia. Blood 2000;96:2317–22.
7. Klein C, Grudzien M, Appaswamy G, et al. HAX1 deficiency causes autosomal recessive severe congenital neutropenia (Kostmann disease). Nat Genet 2007; 39:86–92.
8. Skokowa J, Cario G, Uenalan M, et al. LEF-1 is crucial for neutrophil granulocytopoiesis and its expression is severely reduced in congenital neutropenia. Nat Med 2006;12:1191–7.
9. Radomska HS, Huettner CS, Zhang P, et al. CCAAT/enhancer binding protein a is a regulatory switch sufficient for induction of granulocytic development from bipotential myeloid progenitors. Mol Cell Biol 1998;18:4301–14.
10. Skokowa J, Welte K. Dysregulation of myeloid-specific transcription factors in congenital neutropenia. Ann N Y Acad Sci 2009;1176:94–100.
11. Friedman AD. Transcriptional control of granulocyte and monocyte development [review]. Oncogene 2007;26:6816–28.
12. Dahl R, Walsh JC, Lancki D, et al. Regulation of macrophage and neutrophil cell fates by the PU.1:C/EBPalpha ratio and granulocyte colony-stimulating factor. Nat Immunol 2003;4:1029–36.
13. Rosenbauer F, Tenen DG. Transcription factors in myeloid development: balancing differentiation with transformation [review]. Nat Rev Immunol 2007;7:105–17.
14. Rosenbauer F, Owens BM, Yu L, et al. Lymphoid cell growth and transformation are suppressed by a key regulatory element of the gene encoding PU.1. Nat Genet 2006;38:27–37.
15. Petropoulos K, Arseni N, Schessl C, et al. A novel role for Lef-1, a central transcription mediator of Wnt signaling, in leukemogenesis. J Exp Med 2008;205: 515–22.
16. Klaus A, Birchmeier W. Wnt signalling and its impact on development and cancer. Nat Rev Cancer 2008;8:387–98.
17. Clevers H. Wnt/beta-catenin signaling in development and disease. Cell 2006; 127:469.

18. Reya T, Clevers H. Wnt signalling in stem cells and cancer. Nature 2005;14: 843–50.
19. Logan CY, Nusse R. The Wnt signaling pathway in development and disease. Annu Rev Cell Dev Biol 2004;20:781–810.
20. Clevers H, Nusse R. Wnt/Beta-catenin signaling and disease. Cell 2012;149: 1192–205.
21. Travis A, Amsterdam A, Belanger C, et al. LEF-1, a gene encoding a lymphoid-specific protein with an HMG domain, regulates T-cell receptor a enhancer function. Genes Dev 1991;5:880–94.
22. Giese K, Kingsley C, Kirshner JR, et al. Assembly and function of a TCR alpha enhancer complex is dependent on LEF-1-induced DNA bending and multiple protein-protein interactions. Genes Dev 1995;9:995–1008.
23. Ross DA, Kadesch T. The notch intracellular domain can function as a coactivator for LEF-1. Mol Cell Biol 2001;21:7537–44.
24. Nawshad A, Hay ED. TGFb3 signaling activates transcription of the LEF1 gene to induce epithelial mesenchymal transformation during mouse palate development. J Cell Biol 2003;163:1291–301.
25. Kitamura D, Kaneko H, Miyagoe Y, et al. Isolation and characterization of a novel human gene expressed specifically in the cells of hematopoietic lineage. Nucleic Acids Res 1989;17:9367–79.
26. Skokowa J, Klimiankou M, Klimenkova O, et al. Interaction between HCLS1, HAX1 and LEF-1 proteins is essential for G-CSF-triggered granulopoiesis. Nat Med 2012;18(10):1550–9.
27. Suzuki Y, Demoliere C, Kitamura D, et al. HAX-1, a novel intracellular protein, localized on mitochondria, directly associates with HS1, a substrate of Src family tyrosine kinases. J Immunol 1997;158:2736–44.
28. van Rossum AG, Schuuring-Scholtes E, van Buuren-van Seggelen V, et al. Comparative genome analysis of cortactin and HS1: the significance of the F-actin binding repeat domain. BMC Genomics 2005;6:15.
29. Huang Y, Burkhardt JK. T-cell-receptor-dependent actin regulatory mechanisms [review]. J Cell Sci 2007;120:723–30.
30. Hao JJ, Carey GB, Zhan X. Syk-mediated tyrosine phosphorylation is required for the association of hematopoietic lineage cell-specific protein 1 with lipid rafts and B cell antigen receptor signalosome complex. J Biol Chem 2004;279:33413–20.
31. Takemoto Y, Furuta M, Sato M, et al. Growth factor receptor-bound protein 2 (Grb2) association with hemopoietic specific protein 1: linkage between Lck and Grb2. J Immunol 1998;161:625–30.
32. Ingley E, Sarna MK, Beaumont JG, et al. HS1 interacts with Lyn and is critical for erythropoietin-induced differentiation of erythroid cells. J Biol Chem 2000;275: 7887–93.
33. Yamanashi Y, Okada M, Semba T, et al. Identification of HS1 protein as a major substrate of protein-tyrosine kinase(s) upon B-cell antigen receptor-mediated signaling. Proc Natl Acad Sci U S A 1993;90:3631–5.
34. Brunati AM, Deana R, Folda A, et al. Thrombin-induced tyrosine phosphorylation of HS1 in human platelets is sequentially catalyzed by Syk and Lyn tyrosine kinases and associated with the cellular migration of the protein. J Biol Chem 2005;280:21029–35.
35. Yamanashi Y, Fukuda T, Nishizumi H, et al. Role of tyrosine phosphorylation of HS1 in B cell antigen receptor-mediated apoptosis. J Exp Med 1997;185:1387–92.
36. Hao JJ, Zhu J, Zhou K, et al. The coiled-coil domain is required for HS1 to bind to F-actin and activate Arp2/3 complex. J Biol Chem 2005;280:37988–94.

37. Elsner J, Roesler J, Emmendörffer A, et al. Abnormal regulation in the signal transduction in neutrophils from patients with severe congenital neutropenia: relation of impaired mobilization of cytosolic free calcium to altered chemotaxis, superoxide anion generation and F-actin content. Exp Hematol 1993;21:38–46.
38. Kahner BN, Dorsam RT, Mada SR, et al. Hematopoietic lineage cell–specific protein 1 (HS1) is a functionally important signaling molecule in platelet activation. Blood 2007;110:2449–56.
39. Zhu QS, Xia L, Mills GB, et al. G-CSF induced reactive oxygen species involves Lyn-PI3-kinase-Akt and contributes to myeloid cell growth. Blood 2006;107:1847–56.
40. Otsuka J, Horiuchi T, Yoshizawa S, et al. Association of a four-amino acid residue insertion polymorphism of the HS1 gene with systemic lupus erythematosus: molecular and functional analysis. Arthritis Rheum 2004;50:871–81.
41. Samal B, Sun Y, Stearns G, et al. Cloning and characterization of the cDNA encoding a novel human pre- B cell colony-enhancing factor. Mol Cell Biol 1994;14:1431–7.
42. van der Veer E, Nong Z, O'Neil C, et al. Pre-B cell colony-enhancing factor regulates NAD+-dependent protein deacetylase activity and promotes vascular smooth muscle cell maturation. Circ Res 2005;97:25–34.
43. Rongvaux A, Shea RJ, Mulks MH, et al. Pre-B cell colony-enhancing factor, whose expression is upregulated in activated lymphocytes, is a nicotinamide phosphoribosyltransferase, a cytosolic enzyme involved in NAD biosynthesis. Eur J Immunol 2002;32:3225–34.
44. Skokowa J, Lan D, Thakur BK, et al. NAMPT is essential for the G-CSF–induced myeloid differentiation via a NAD+–sirtuin-1–dependent pathway. Nat Med 2009;15:151–8.
45. Hirai H, Zhang P, Dayaram T, et al. C/EBPbeta is required for 'emergency' granulopoiesis. Nat Immunol 2006;7:732–9.
46. Allport JR, Lim YC, Shipley JM, et al. Neutrophils from MMP-9- or neutrophil elastase-deficient mice show no defect in transendothelial migration under flow in vitro. J Leukoc Biol 2002;71:821–8.
47. Sera Y, Kawaguchi H, Nakamura K, et al. A comparison of the defective granulopoiesis in childhood cyclic neutropenia and in severe congenital neutropenia. Haematologica 2005;90:1032–41.
48. Nakamura K, Kobayashi M, Konishi N, et al. Defects of granulopoiesis in patients with severe congenital neutropenia. Hiroshima J Med Sci 2002;51:63–74.
49. Konishi N, Kobayashi M, Miyagawa S, et al. Defective proliferation of primitive myeloid progenitor cells in patients with severe congenital neutropenia. Blood 1999;94:4077–83.
50. Köllner I, Sodeik B, Schreek S, et al. Mutations in neutrophil elastase causing congenital neutropenia lead to cytoplasmic protein accumulation and induction of the unfolded protein response. Blood 2006;108:493–500.
51. Grenda DS, Murakami M, Ghatak J, et al. Mutations of the ELA2 gene found in patients with severe congenital neutropenia induce the unfolded protein response and cellular apoptosis. Blood 2007;110:4179–87.
52. Nanua S, Murakami M, Xia J, et al. Activation of the unfolded protein response is associated with impaired granulopoiesis in transgenic mice expressing mutant Elane. Blood 2011;117:3539–47.
53. Skokowa J, Fobiwe JP, Dan L, et al. Neutrophil elastase is severely downregulated in severe congenital neutropenia independent of ELA2 or HAX1 mutations but dependent on LEF-1. Blood 2009;114:3044–51.

54. Takahashi H, Nukiwa T, Basset P, et al. Myelomonocytic cell lineage expression of the neutrophil elastase gene. J Biol Chem 1988;263:2543–7.

55. El Ouriaghli F, Fujiwara H, Melenhorst JJ, et al. Neutrophil elastase enzymatically antagonizes the in vitro action of G-CSF: implications for the regulation of granulopoiesis. Blood 2003;101:1752–8.

56. Hunter MG, Druhan LJ, Massullo PR, et al. Proteolytic cleavage of granulocyte colony-stimulating factor and its receptor by neutrophil elastase induces growth inhibition and decreased cell surface expression of the granulocyte colony-stimulating factor receptor. Am J Hematol 2003;74:149–55.

57. Rao RM, Betz TV, Lamont DJ, et al. Elastase release by transmigrating neutrophils deactivates endothelialbound SDF-1alpha and attenuates subsequent T lymphocyte transendothelial migration. J Exp Med 2004;200:713–24.

58. Levesque JP, Takamatsu Y, Nilsson SK, et al. Vascular cell adhesion mole- cule-1 (CD106) is cleaved by neutrophil proteases in the bone marrow following hematopoietic progenitor cell mobilization by granulocyte colony-stimulating factor. Blood 2001;98:1289–97.

59. Levesque JP, Hendy J, Winkler IG, et al. Granulocyte colony-stimulating factor induces the release in the bone marrow of proteases that cleave c-KIT receptor (CD117) from the surface of hematopoietic progenitor cells. Exp Hematol 2003; 31:109–17.

60. Levesque JP, Hendy J, Takamatsu Y, et al. Mobilization by either cyclophosphamide or granulocyte colony-stimulating factor transforms the bone marrow into a highly proteolytic environment. Exp Hematol 2002;30:440–9.

61. Jin F, Zhai Q, Qiu L, et al. Degradation of BM SDF-1 by MMP-9: the role in G-CSF-induced hematopoietic stem/progenitor cell mobilization. Bone Marrow Transplant 2008;42:581–8.

62. Valenzuela-Fernandez A, Planchenault T, Baleux F, et al. Leukocyte elastase negatively regulates stromal cell-derived factor-1 (SDF-1)/CXCR4 binding and functions by amino-terminal processing of SDF-1 and CXCR4. J Biol Chem 2002;277:15677–89.

63. Lapidot T, Petit I. Current understanding of stem cell mobilization: the roles of chemokines, proteolytic enzymes, adhesion molecules, cytokines, and stromal cells. Exp Hematol 2002;30:973–81.

64. Levesque JP, Hendy J, Takamatsu Y, et al. Disruption of the CXCR4/CXCL12 chemotactic interaction during hematopoietic stem cell mobilization induced by GCSF or cyclophosphamide. J Clin Invest 2003;111:187–96.

65. Rosenberg PS, Zeidler C, Bolyard AA, et al. Stable long-term risk of leukaemia in patients with severe congenital neutropenia maintained on G-CSF therapy. Br J Haematol 2010;150:196–9.

66. Rauprich P, Kasper B, Tidow N, et al. The protein tyrosine kinase JAK2 is activated in neutrophils from patients with severe congenital neutropenia. Blood 1995;86:4500–5.

67. Flores-Morales A, Fernández L, Rico-Bautista E, et al. Endoplasmic reticulum stress prolongs GH-induced Janus kinase (JAK2)/signal transducer and activator of transcription (STAT5) signaling pathway. Mol Endocrinol 2001;15:1471–83.

68. Kato Y, Iwama A, Tadokoro Y, et al. Selective activation of STAT5 unveils its role in stem cell self-renewal in normal and leukemic hematopoiesis. J Exp Med 2005; 202:169–79.

69. Thakur BK, Dittrich T, Chandra P, et al. Involvement of p53 in the cytotoxic activity of the NAMPT inhibitor FK866 in myeloid leukemic cells. Int J Cancer 2012;131.

70. Thakur BK, Lippka Y, Dittrich T, et al. NAMPT pathway is involved in the FOXO3a-mediated regulation of GADD45A expression. Biochem Biophys Res Commun 2012;420:714–20.
71. Dan L, Klimenkova O, Klimiankou M, et al. The role of sirtuin 2 activation by nicotinamide phosphoribosyltransferase in the aberrant proliferation and survival of myeloid leukemia cells. Haematologica 2012;97:551–9.

Chronic Granulomatous Disease

Steven M. Holland, MD

KEYWORDS

- Chronic granulomatous disease • Gene defects • NADPH oxidase • Immune defect
- Inflammatory bowel disease

KEY POINTS

- Chronic granulomatous disease (CGD) is a single gene defect that can be reconstituted in vitro and does not require complete correction to be effective, as proven by the normal lives of many X-linked carriers, and by the stable chimeras generated in some transplant protocols.
- Unlike the case with severe combined immunodeficiency, corrected CGD cells do not have a growth or survival advantage in the marrow or tissue. Therefore, selection and augmentation of those cells is difficult.
- Nicotinamide adenine dinucleotide phosphate (NADPH) oxidase is active outside the neutrophil, such as in nuclear factor κβ signaling, liver damage from carcinogens, and the arterial vasculature.
- NADPH oxidase somatic and hematopoietic activity is involved in strokes and pulmonary vascular permeability. NADPH contributes to long-term potentiation of memory and may be related to IQ.
- NADPH oxidase is clearly active in many more sites than just phagocytes, suggesting that CGD is more complex and can teach about more than just infections and bone marrow transplants alone.

Chronic granulomatous disease (CGD) was first described in 1954[1] and 1957[2] as recurrent infections occurring in the setting of hypergammaglobulinemia, as opposed to the disease then recently recognized by Bruton,[3] in which infections were associated with hypogammaglobulinemia. The disease was not well characterized until 1959,[4] when it was initially termed *fatal granulomatous disease of childhood*, but it is now simply referred to as *chronic granulomatous disease*. Originally thought to be only an X-linked disease, its recognition in girls in 1968 also led to the determination of autosomal recessive forms.[5] Over almost 60 years, CGD has evolved from a disease of early fatality to one of effective management with high survival.[6] CGD is a paradigm

This work supported by the Division of Intramural Research, National Institute of Allergy and Infectious Diseases, National Institutes of Health.
Laboratory of Clinical Infectious Diseases, National Institute of Allergy and Infectious Diseases, National Institutes of Health, CRC B3-4141, MSC 1684, Bethesda, MD 20892-1684, USA
E-mail address: smh@nih.gov

Hematol Oncol Clin N Am 27 (2013) 89–99
http://dx.doi.org/10.1016/j.hoc.2012.11.002
0889-8588/13/$ – see front matter Published by Elsevier Inc.

for nonlymphoid primary immune defects, and has guided elucidation of oxygen metabolism in the phagocyte, vasculature, and brain.[7] It has been in the forefront of the development of antimicrobial prophylaxis before the advent of advanced HIV and before its routine use in neutropenia.[8] It has been an attractive target for gene therapy and bone marrow transplantation for nonmalignant diseases. Therefore, CGD is worthy of attention for its historical interest and because it is a disease for which expert management is imperative.

Multiple separate proteins contribute to the intact nicotinamide adenine dinucleotide phosphate (NADPH) oxidase, mutations in 5 of which lead to the single syndrome of CGD. NADPH oxidase catalyzes the transfer of an electron from cytoplasmic NADPH to molecular oxygen (6; OMIM# 306400, 233690, 233700, 233710, 601488), thereby oxidizing NADPH and leading to the name *NADPH oxidase*. Although impairments of the NADPH oxidase typically present as phagocyte defects, in fact only gp91^{phox} is relatively phagocyte-specific, whereas the other autosomal components are also expressed elsewhere.[7] The components are broken into membrane-bound (cytochrome b558, composed of gp91^{phox} and p22^{phox}) and cytosolic (p47^{phox}, p67^{phox}, and p40^{phox}) structures. The subunits gp91^{phox} and p22^{phox} require each other for expression in the phagocyte; however, because p22^{phox} is expressed in other tissues and gp91^{phox} is not, p22^{phox} and the other members of the NADPH oxidase join with other partners in the other tissues, which are other members of the *Nox* family of proteins. Therefore, individuals who have autosomal recessive forms of CGD may also have other subtle abnormalities, such as vascular disease and diabetes in p47^{phox}-deficient CGD or perhaps inflammatory bowel disease in p40^{phox}-deficient CGD.[9]

Activation of the NADPH oxidase is a carefully choreographed process.[6] On cellular activation, such as ingestion of bacteria of fungi, the cytosolic components p47^{phox} and p67^{phox} are phosphorylated and bind tightly together. The secondary (specific) granules, which contain the cytochrome complex (gp91^{phox} and p22^{phox}) fuse with the phagolysosome, followed by the primary (azurophilic) granules, which contain the antibacterial peptides neutrophil elastase and cathepsin G. This process embeds the cytochrome in the wall of the phagolysosome and the antibacterial peptides inside it. The cytoplasmic complex of p47^{phox} and p67^{phox} in association with p40^{phox} and RAC2 combine with the cytochrome to form the intact NADPH oxidase, which is oriented into the internal aspect of the phagolysosome (this process can also occur on the plasma membrane focused outside the cell). An electron is then taken from cytoplasmic NADPH and donated to molecular oxygen inside the phagolysosome, leading to the formation of superoxide. In the presence of superoxide dismutase, this is converted to hydrogen peroxide, which, in the presence of myeloperoxidase and chlorine in the phagolysosome, is converted to bleach. Although the metabolites of superoxide themselves can contribute to bacterial killing, the generation of superoxide has broader implications.[10] With the generation of superoxide, a charge is imparted to the phagolysosome that is rectified by the rapid influx of potassium ions.[11] This potassium influx leads to activation of the now-intraphagosomal peptides, which mediate microbial killing.[10,11] Therefore, reactive oxidants are working more as intracellular signaling molecules, leading to activation of other nonoxidative pathways in addition to causing killing directly. Thus, a spectrum of microbicidal activity can be regulated by NADPH oxidase activity, rather than distinct oxidative and nonoxidative pathways and mechanisms.

In addition to activation of intracellular antimicrobial peptides, the NADPH oxidase is required to activate neutrophil extracellular traps (NETs), complex assemblies of DNA and antimicrobial peptides released from apoptotic neutrophils.[12] Repair of the NADPH oxidase system with gene therapy in a patient with X-linked CGD led to reconstitution of NET function, proving that NET formation is impaired in CGD and dependent on NADPH function.[13]

Mutations in all of the 5 structural genes of the NADPH oxidase have been found to cause CGD. Mutations in gp91^{phox} account for approximately 65% of cases, mutations in p47^{phox} account for approximately 25%, and the remainder are divided between p67^{phox} and p22^{phox} [6,14]; one case of p40^{phox} deficiency has been reported.[9] No autosomal dominant cases of CGD have been reported. A large voluntary retrospective study in the United States and Europe suggested rates of CGD of around 1 in 200,000 to 1 in 250,000 live births.[14,15] Rates in other countries vary depending on the ethnic practices and degrees of intermarriage: Sweden 1 in 450,000; Japan 1 in 300,000; Israeli Jews 1 in 218,000; Israeli Arabs 1 in 111,000.[16] However, the relative rates of X-linked compared with recessive CGD are distinct. In many countries with high rates of consanguineous marriage, recessive CGD rates exceed X-linked rates.[15,16] Clinically, X-linked gp91^{phox}-deficient CGD is more severe with earlier presentation and diagnosis, and more severe infections and earlier death than the p47^{phox}-deficient form.[14,15]

Mechanistically, the level of residual superoxide production determines survival, at least in X-linked CGD.[17] The rates of long-term survival are higher in those patients with X-linked CGD with higher residual superoxide production and lower in those with lower production. Molecularly, this is caused by the ability of the mutant protein to support superoxide production. Thus, mutations that lead to no protein production (nonsense mutations, deletions, certain splice defects) support no residual superoxide production and have the lowest level of survival. In contrast, those mutations that permit protein production and superoxide generation (missense mutations before amino acid 310 except histidine 222) are associated with higher survival rates. However, mutations at or beyond amino acid 310 are unable to support superoxide production, presumably because of the strict structural requirements of the intracellular domain of gp91^{phox} for the binding of NADPH and flavin adenine dinucleotide (FAD).[17]

Infections of the lung, skin, lymph nodes, and liver are the most frequent first manifestations of CGD.[6,15] In North America, most infections in CGD are from *Staphylococcus aureus, Burkholderia cepacia* complex*, Serratia marcescens, Nocardia* spp, and *Aspergillus* spp.[6] In other parts of the world *Salmonella, Bacille Calmette–Guérin* (BCG), and tuberculosis are also important.[15,16] Patients with CGD tend to develop severe localized BCG rather than disseminated BCGosis. Trimethoprim/sulfamethoxazole prophylaxis has reduced the frequency of bacterial infections in general and staphylococcal infections in particular. On prophylaxis, staphylococcal infections are essentially confined to the liver and cervical lymph nodes.[6] Staphylococcal liver abscesses encountered in CGD are dense, caseous, and difficult to drain, and previously required surgery in almost all cases.[18] However, recent studies have shown that the combination of corticosteroids and antibiotics alone are highly effective in CGD liver abscesses, allowing cure of liver abscesses without surgery.[19,20] Until recently fungal infections, typically because of *Aspergillus* spp, were the leading cause of mortality in CGD.[14,15] The advent of highly active antifungal therapy with the orally active azole antifungals itraconazole, voriconazole, and posaconazole has changed the face of fungal infections in CGD. Mortality from *A fumigatus* infection in CGD is now uncommon, and therefore mortality overall is diminished.[21] However, the non-*fumigatus Aspergillus* spp, and some species of fungi other than *Aspergillus* remain difficult to treat and important contributors to mortality.[22,23]

Overall survival in CGD is now thought to be approximately 90%, stretching well into adulthood.[24] Patients diagnosed before the advent of antifungal azole agents had different outcomes, reflected by the poor survival of patients into their 30s and 40s in some series.[14,15] Since the introduction of itraconazole in the late 1990s, its proof in antifungal prophylaxis in 2003,[25] and the introduction of more active antifungals and antibacterials, mortality in CGD has plunged.[24,26] Access to expert care is clearly important, as shown by a Japanese study with a 90% survival rate for patients followed up at single center.[27] Similarly, Mouy and colleagues[28] found an 8-year survival rate of 70.5% for children born before 1978 but a 92.9% survival rate for those born later. Before the introduction of oral antifungals Winkelstein and colleagues[14] reported X-linked CGD mortality of approximately 5% per year, compared with 2% per year for the autosomal recessive varieties. van den Berg and colleagues[15] found a 23% mortality in X-linked CGD and a 15% rate of mortality in autosomal recessive CGD over almost 50 years of European survey. Therefore, overall mortality from infection in CGD has been significant but will continue to improve with better therapies.

The morbidity of recurrent infections and inflammation, with their associated end-organ damage and their impact on the child and family, is a major issue. Several large studies found similar rates of infection of around 0.3 per year.[24,26] That is, most patients are still experiencing at least one severe infection every 3 to 4 years, whether bacterial or fungal. The persistence of this rate may reflect a minimum inescapable environmental exposure, or the complexity of maintaining long-term prophylaxis over a lifetime with a disease that is only intermittently reinforced.

CGD is remarkable because of its very narrow but profound spectrum of infection susceptibility. B cepacia complex organisms are common causes of pneumonia and, infrequently, sepsis.[29] The closely related B gladioli has also been described in CGD.[30] Chromobacterium violaceum is found in brackish waters, such as those around the Gulf of Mexico in the United States, and causes sepsis in CGD.[31] Francisella philomiragia causes sepsis in CGD and is also found in brackish waters, such as the Chesapeake Bay, Long Island Sound, and around Nova Scotia.[32] Granulibacter bethesdensis is a novel gram-negative rod that causes chronic necrotizing lymphadenitis and can cause sepsis in CGD.[33] It can have latent and active phases, similar to tuberculosis, and has been identified in the United States, Panama, and Spain, suggesting wide distribution. Although the rate of seropositivity for this organism is approximately 50% in patients with CGD, most of whom have not had recognized infections, this rate is around 25% in patients without CGD, suggesting broad exposure and the possibility of a clinical syndrome yet to be identified.[34]

Fungal infections are critically important to recognize in CGD. Several are characteristic of CGD and virtually never encountered in other diseases: A nidulans, Paecilomyces variotii and P lilacinus, and Neosartorya udagawae. These organisms are highly pathogenic in those infected with CGD but not in any other patient group, including transplant recipients.[35] In contrast to these filamentous molds that are virtually pathognomonic for CGD, the endemic dimorphic mold infections histoplasmosis, blastomycosis, and coccidioidomycosis do not occur in CGD, nor does cryptococcosis. Mucormycosis occurs in CGD but only in the setting of significant immunosuppression.[36] The molecular identification of infection should be vigorously pursued in patients with CGD, especially for fungal infections, because the identification of a non-fumigatus Aspergillus infection should prompt early consideration of therapeutic surgery.[37]

Fungal elements elicit an exuberant inflammatory response in CGD regardless of whether they are live or dead.[38] Mulch pneumonitis refers to acute inhalational exposure to aerosolized decayed organic matter, such as mulch, hay, or dead leaves.[39] The clinical presentation is stereotypic and dramatic: a previously well child or adult spreads mulch, turns compost, or clears moldy leaves, inhaling numerous fungal spores and hyphae; 1 to 10 days later a syndrome similar to hypersensitivity pneumonitis begins with fever and dyspnea; chest radiographs show diffuse interstitial infiltrates; bronchoscopy is usually uninformative but may yield *Aspergillus*; lung biopsy shows acute inflammation with necrotizing granulomata and fungi. The most successful treatments of this syndrome have been with simultaneous antifungals for the infection and steroids for the inflammation.[39] The authors typically institute meropenem, voriconazole, and prednisone for this syndrome, because steroids seem to be crucial for reducing inflammation and allowing independent ventilation. This syndrome should be considered in all cases of *Aspergillus* pneumonitis, especially with acute onset and hypoxia, and therefore implies CGD as the underlying diagnosis. This syndrome occurs in patients with known CGD but also may be the presentation for disease, even in adults.

Inflammation in CGD is most prominent in the gastrointestinal and genitourinary tracts. Esophageal, jejunal, ileal, cecal, rectal, and perirectal involvement with granulomata mimicking Crohn disease have been described.[40,41] Functional gastric outlet obstruction may be the initial presentation of CGD. In a large survey of patients with CGD followed at the National Institutes of Health, 43% of those with X-linked CGD had symptomatic, biopsy-proven inflammatory bowel disease (IBD), compared with only 11% of $p47^{phox}$-deficient patients.[40] However, growth rates were equally diminished to less than the mean in IBD-affected and unaffected patients. Whether the mild growth retardation seen in most patients with CGD was from IBD in all cases, or from some other CGD-associated feature of the disease is unknown, because biopsies were only performed in symptomatic patients. Growth and growth rates in CGD recovered after bone marrow transplantation, regardless of antecedent IBD.[42] Although IBD may involve any part of the gastrointestinal tract in patients with CGD, perirectal disease is especially common.[41]

Treatment of CGD IBD is often long-term and difficult, and the disease is prone to relapse. Steroids are effective but may cause growth retardation, osteoporosis, and infection risk. However, at the doses typically used in CGD for maintenance, infections are rarely an issue. In contrast, although tumor necrosis factor (TNF)-α–blocking agents are highly effective and rapidly suppress bowel symptoms, they confer a high risk of infection and death and should be carefully avoided in patients with CGD.[43] TNF-α inhibitors predispose to characteristic CGD pathogens, only more severe episodes. The authors' current practice is to initiate therapy for proven IBD in CGD with prednisone at 1 mg/kg/d for 1 to 2 weeks and then slowly taper to 0.1 to 0.25 mg/kg/d over 1 to 2 months. Sometimes prednisone can be stopped in children, but the relapse rate is very high, and re-treatment typically requires reinitiation of the higher dose. Therefore, after the first recurrence or relapse the authors usually add an antimetabolite, such as azathioprine (Imuran), along with salicylic acid derivatives. Local treatments such as steroid enemas and rectal creams are also highly effective.

Liver involvement in CGD is pronounced and important. Liver abscesses occur in approximately 35% of patients and until recently have been difficult to treat without surgery.[18] With surgery, cure of liver abscess is common, but unfortunately so is reinfection, typically with a different organism from the previous one. Whether certain patients with CGD are simply predisposed to liver abscesses or having had a previous liver abscess alters hepatic architecture and blood flow in a way that makes subsequent infection more likely remains unclear. High rates of portal venopathy and nodular regenerative hyperplasia may contribute to portal hypertension, splenomegaly, and splenic sequestration.[44] This latter point is noteworthy, because the decline in platelet count is linked to splenomegaly and is also a strong predictor of mortality in CGD.[45] Chronic drug effects, liver enzyme elevations, and recurrent infections are obvious risks for liver dysfunction. In this regard, whether the predilection for recurrent liver abscesses is partly caused by surgery, with its hepatic scarring and altered blood flow, is unclear. However, avoiding surgery when possible seems prudent, and the recent demonstration of the effectiveness of steroids and antibiotics alone in the resolution of liver abscess offers an alternative treatment.[20]

Genitourinary manifestations of CGD are also common and include bladder granulomata, ureteral obstruction, and urinary tract infection, typically in those with gp91^{phox} and p22^{phox} deficiencies.[46] Eosinophilic cystitis has also been described in CGD.[47] Genitourinary complications are also highly steroid responsive. Inflammatory masses in CGD can mimic tumors and should be considered.[48]

The diagnosis of CGD is usually made by direct measurement of superoxide production, ferricytochrome c reduction, chemiluminescence, nitroblue tetrazolium (NBT) reduction, or dihydrorhodamine oxidation (DHR). DHR is preferable because of its relative ease of use, its ability to distinguish X-linked from autosomal patterns of CGD on flow cytometry, its sensitivity to even very low numbers of functional neutrophils, and its utility in predicting the residual superoxide activity of the patient's neutrophils.[17,49] The 2 conditions known to give a falsely abnormal DHR are myeloperoxidase deficiency[50] and SAPHO syndrome.[51] In myeloperoxidase deficiency, the DHR tracing can look like that of X-linked CGD, whereas the NBT and ferricytochrome c results are normal. This finding is attributed to intracellular (DHR) compared with extracellular (NBT) superoxide release and dye activation. Glucose 6-phosphate dehydrogenase (G6PD) deficiency may also lead to a decreased respiratory burst and increased susceptibility to bacterial infections.[52] However, G6PD deficiency is most often associated with some degree of hemolytic anemia, whereas CGD is not.

Female carriers of X-linked CGD have 2 populations of phagocytes: 1 that produces superoxide and 1 that does not, yielding a characteristic mosaic pattern on oxidative testing. Infections are infrequent unless the normal neutrophils are less than 10%, and even then are uncommon. However, cases of severe skewing of X-chromosome inactivation have been reported, in which women have virtually no detectable normal cells; these carriers are at risk for CGD-type infections.[53] Reports suggest that the balance of wild-type to mutant cells may vary over time in the same woman, but this has not been rigorously proven, as likely as it may seem.[53] Discoid lupus erythematosus–like lesions, aphthous ulcers, and photosensitive rashes have been seen in gp91^{phox} carriers. Similarly, screening of patients with discoid lupus erythematosus detected a significant number of previously unsuspected CGD carriers.[54–56]

Immunoblot and flow cytometry can be used to infer the specific genotype, but molecular determination of specific mutations is necessary for prenatal diagnosis. A robust genotype/phenotype correlation has been shown for mutations that permit residual superoxide production compared with those that do not.[17] Male sex, earlier age at presentation, and increased severity of disease suggest X-linked disease, but these are only rough guides. The precise gene defect should probably be determined in all cases, because it is a strong predictor of survival. Autosomal recessive p47^{phox}-deficient CGD has a significantly better prognosis than X-linked disease.[14,15,17]

Effective management of CGD is predicated on prophylactic antibiotics and antifungals and interferon (IFN)-γ, along with management of acute infections as they occur. Prophylactic trimethoprim/sulfamethoxazole (5 mg/kg/d trimethoprim divided twice daily) reduces the frequency of major infections from approximately once every year to once every 3.5 years, reducing staphylococcal and skin infections without increasing in the frequency of serious fungal infections in CGD.[57] Itraconazole prophylaxis prevents fungal infections in CGD (100 mg daily for patients aged <13 y or weighing <50 kg; 200 mg daily for those aged >13 y or weighing >50 kg).[25] IFN-γ was shown in a large, multinational, multicenter, placebo-controlled study to reduce the number and severity of infections in CGD by 70% compared with placebo regardless of inheritance pattern, sex, or use of prophylactic antibiotics.[58] Systemic IFN-γ also augmented neutrophil activity against *Aspergillus* conidia in vitro.[59] Furthermore, in a study of IFN-γ in CGD mice, infections were reduced.[60] However, a retrospective Italian study detected no benefit to the addition of IFN-γ beyond that attributed to antibacterial and antifungals alone.[24] Long-term follow-up of the large prospective trials suggests sustained benefit.[26] The authors use trimethoprim/sulfamethoxazole, itraconazole, and IFN-γ (50 μg/m²) in the treatment of CGD.

Bone marrow transplantation can lead to stable remission of CGD. Regimens ranging from full myeloablation to nonmyeloablative conditioning lead to cure of CGD.[42,61,62] Even in the setting of refractory fungal infection, bone marrow transplantation has been effective.[63] Nonmyeloablative transplants in CGD have been more successful in children than in adults.[64] Although bone marrow transplantation is an attractive option for the definitive cure of CGD, survival without bone marrow transplantation is roughly comparable, but attended by continuing CGD morbidities, such as bowel disease and mildly reduced growth.

CGD is a group of single gene defects that can be reconstituted in vitro and does not require complete correction to be effective, as proven by the normal lives of many X-linked carriers, and by the stable chimeras generated in some transplant protocols.[65] Unlike the case with severe combined immunodeficiency, corrected CGD cells do not have a growth or survival advantage in the marrow or tissue. Therefore, in vivo selection and augmentation of those cells is difficult.

NADPH oxidase is active outside the neutrophil, such as in nuclear factor κβ signaling, liver damage from carcinogens, and the arterial vasculature.[66–68] NADPH oxidase somatic and hematopoietic activity is involved in strokes and pulmonary vascular permeability.[69] NADPH contributes to long-term potentiation of memory[70] and may be related to IQ.[71] Therefore, NADPH oxidase is clearly active in many more sites than just phagocytes, suggesting that CGD is more complex and can teach about more than just infections and bone marrow transplants alone.

REFERENCES

1. Janeway CA, Craig J, Davidson M, et al. Hypergammaglobulinemia associated with severe, recurrent and chronic non-specific infection. Am J Dis Child 1954; 88:388–92.
2. Berendes H, Bridges RA, Good RA. A fatal granulomatous disease of childhood: the clinical study of a new syndrome. Minn Med 1957;40:309.
3. Bruton OC. Agammaglobulinemia. Pediatrics 1952;9(6):722–8.
4. Bridges RA, Berendes H, Good RA. A fatal granulomatous disease of childhood. Am J Dis Child 1959;97:387.
5. Azimi PH, Bodenbender JG, Hintz RL, et al. Chronic granulomatous disease in three female siblings. JAMA 1968;206:2865–70.
6. Segal BH, Leto TL, Gallin JI, et al. Genetic, biochemical, and clinical features of chronic granulomatous disease. Medicine (Baltimore) 2000;79:170–200.
7. Ushio-Fukai M. Localizing NADPH oxidase-derived ROS. Sci STKE 2006;349:re8.
8. Freeman AF, Holland SM. Antimicrobial prophylaxis for primary immunodeficiencies. Curr Opin Allergy Clin Immunol 2009;9(6):525–30.
9. Matute JD, Arias AA, Wright NA, et al. A new genetic subgroup of chronic granulomatous disease with autosomal recessive mutations in p40 phox and selective defects in neutrophil NADPH oxidase activity. Blood 2009;114(15):3309–15.

10. Tkalcevic J, Novelli M, Phylactides M, et al. Impaired immunity and enhanced resistance to endotoxin in the absence of neutrophil elastase and cathepsin G. Immunity 2000;12(2):201–10.

11. Reeves EP, Lu H, Jacobs HL, et al. Killing activity of neutrophils is mediated through activation of proteases by K+ flux. Nature 2002;416:291–7.

12. Fuchs TA, Abed U, Goosmann C, et al. Novel cell death program leads to neutrophil extracellular traps. J Cell Biol 2007;176(2):231–41.

13. Bianchi M, Hakkim A, Brinkmann V, et al. Restoration of NET formation by gene therapy in CGD controls aspergillosis. Blood 2009;114(13):2619–22.

14. Winkelstein JA, Marino MC, Johnston RB Jr, et al. Chronic granulomatous disease. Report on a national registry of 368 patients. Medicine (Baltimore) 2000;79:155–69.

15. van den Berg JM, van Koppen E, Ahlin A, et al. Chronic granulomatous disease: the European experience. PLoS One 2009;4(4):e5234. http://dx.doi.org/10.1371/journal.pone.0005234.

16. Wolach B, Gavrieli R, de Boer M, et al. Chronic granulomatous disease in Israel: clinical, functional and molecular studies of 38 patients. Clin Immunol 2008;129:103–14.

17. Kuhns DB, Alvord WG, Heller T, et al. Long term survival and residual NADPH oxidase function in chronic granulomatous disease. N Engl J Med 2010;363(27):2600–10.

18. Lublin M, Bartlett DL, Danforth DN, et al. Hepatic abscess in patients with chronic granulomatous disease. Ann Surg 2002;235:383–91.

19. Yamazaki-Nakashimada MA, Stiehm ER, Pietropaolo-Cienfuegos D, et al. Corticosteroid therapy for refractory infections in chronic granulomatous disease: case reports and review of the literature. Ann Allergy Asthma Immunol 2006;97:257–61.

20. Leiding JW, Freeman AF, Marciano BE, et al. Corticosteroid therapy for liver abscess in chronic granulomatous disease. Clin Infect Dis 2011;54:694–700.

21. Blumental S, Mouy R, Mahlaoui N, et al. Invasive mold infections in chronic granulomatous disease: a 25-year retrospective survey. Clin Infect Dis 2011;53:e159–69.

22. Vinh DC, Shea YR, Sugui JA, et al. Invasive aspergillosis due to Neosartorya udagawae. Clin Infect Dis 2009;49(1):102–11.

23. Vinh DC, Shea YR, Jones PA, et al. Chronic invasive aspergillosis caused by Aspergillus viridinutans. Emerg Infect Dis 2009;15(8):1292–4.

24. Martire B, Rondelli R, Soresina A, et al. Clinical features, long-term follow-up and outcome of a large cohort of patients with Chronic Granulomatous Disease: an Italian multicenter study. Clin Immunol 2008;126:155–64.

25. Gallin JI, Alling DW, Malech HL, et al. Itraconazole to prevent fungal infections in chronic granulomatous disease. N Engl J Med 2003;348:2416–22.

26. Marciano BE, Wesley R, De Carlo ES, et al. Long-term interferon-gamma therapy for patients with chronic granulomatous disease. Clin Infect Dis 2004;39:692–9.

27. Kobayashi S, Murayama S, Takanashi S, et al. Clinical features and prognoses of 23 patients with chronic granulomatous disease followed for 21 years by a single hospital in Japan. Eur J Pediatr 2008;167:1389–94.

28. Mouy R, Fischer A, Vilmer E, et al. Incidence, severity and prevention of infections in chronic granulomatous disease. J Pediatr 1989;114:555–60.

29. Greenberg DE, Goldberg JB, Stock F, et al. Recurrent Burkholderia infection in patients with chronic granulomatous disease: 11-year experience at a large referral center. Clin Infect Dis 2009;48(11):1577–9.

30. Ross JP, Holland SM, Gill VJ, et al. Severe Burkholderia (Pseudomonas) gladioli infection in chronic granulomatous disease: report of two successfully treated cases. Clin Infect Dis 1995;21:1291–3.
31. Sirinavin S, Techasaensiri C, Benjaponpitak S, et al. Invasive Chromobacterium violaceum infection in children: case report and review. Pediatr Infect Dis J 2005;24:559–61.
32. Mailman TL, Schmidt MH. Francisella philomiragia adenitis and pulmonary nodules in a child with chronic granulomatous disease. Can J Infect Dis Med Microbiol 2005;16:245–8.
33. Greenberg DE, Shoffner AR, Zelazny AM, et al. Recurrent Granulibacter bethesdensis infections and chronic granulomatous disease. Emerg Infect Dis 2010; 16(9):1341–8.
34. Greenberg DE, Shoffner AR, Marshall-Batty KR, et al. Serologic reactivity to the emerging pathogen granulibacter bethesdensis. J Infect Dis 2012;206: 943–51.
35. Falcone EL, Holland SM. Invasive fungal infection in chronic granulomatous disease: insights into pathogenesis and management. Curr Opin Infect Dis 2012;25:658–69.
36. Vinh DC, Freeman AF, Shea YR, et al. Mucormycosis in chronic granulomatous disease: association with iatrogenic immunosuppression. J Allergy Clin Immunol 2009;123(6):1411–3.
37. Sugui JA, Vinh DC, Nardone G, et al. Neosartorya udagawae (Aspergillus udagawae), an emerging agent of aspergillosis: how different is it from aspergillus fumigatus? J Clin Microbiol 2010;48(1):220–8.
38. Morgenstern DE, Gifford MA, Li LL, et al. Absence of respiratory burst in X-linked chronic granulomatous disease mice leads to abnormalities in both host defense and inflammatory response to Aspergillus fumigatus. J Exp Med 1997;185: 207–18.
39. Siddiqui S, Anderson VL, Hilligoss DM, et al. Fulminant mulch pneumonitis: an emergency presentation of chronic granulomatous disease. Clin Infect Dis 2007;45:673–81.
40. Marciano BE, Rosenzweig SD, Kleiner DE, et al. Gastrointestinal involvement in chronic granulomatous disease. Pediatrics 2004;114:462–8.
41. Marks DJ, Miyagi K, Rahman FZ, et al. Inflammatory bowel disease in CGD reproduces the clinicopathological features of Crohn's disease. Am J Gastroenterol 2009;104:117–24.
42. Soncini E, Slatter MA, Jones LB, et al. Unrelated donor and HLA-identical sibling haematopoietic stem cell transplantation cure chronic granulomatous disease with good long-term outcome and growth. Br J Haematol 2009;145:73–83.
43. Uzel G, Orange JS, Poliak N, et al. Complications of tumor necrosis factor-α blockade in chronic granulomatous disease-related colitis. Clin Infect Dis 2010; 51(12):1429–34.
44. Hussain N, Feld JJ, Kleiner DE, et al. Hepatic abnormalities in patients with chronic granulomatous disease. Hepatology 2007;45:675–83.
45. Feld JJ, Hussain N, Wright EC, et al. Hepatic involvement and portal hypertension predict mortality in chronic granulomatous disease. Gastroenterology 2008;134: 1917–26.
46. Walther MM, Malech HL, Berman A, et al. The urologic manifestations of chronic granulomatous disease. J Urol 1992;147:1314–8.
47. Barese CN, Podestá M, Litvak E, et al. Recurrent eosinophilic cystitis in a child with chronic granulomatous disease. J Pediatr Hematol Oncol 2004;26:209–12.

48. Hauck F, Heine S, Beier R, et al. Chronic granulomatous disease (CGD) mimicking neoplasms: a suspected mediastinal teratoma unmasking as thymic granulomas due to X-linked CGD, and 2 related cases. J Pediatr Hematol Oncol 2008;30:877–80.
49. Elloumi HZ, Holland SM. Diagnostic assays for chronic granulomatous disease and other neutrophil disorders. Methods Mol Biol 2007;412:505–23.
50. Mauch L, Lun A, O'Gorman MR, et al. Chronic granulomatous disease (CGD) and complete myeloperoxidase deficiency both yield strongly reduced dihydrorhod-amine 123 test signals but can be easily discerned in routine testing for CGD. Clin Chem 2007;53:890–6.
51. Ferguson PJ, Lokuta MA, El-Shanti HI, et al. Neutrophil dysfunction in a family with a SAPHO syndrome-like phenotype. Arthritis Rheum 2008;58:3264–9.
52. Roos D, van Zwieten R, Wijnen JT, et al. Molecular basis and enzymatic proper-ties of glucose-6-phosphate dehydrogenase volendam, leading to chronic nonspherocytic anemia, granulocyte dysfunction, and increased susceptibility to infections. Blood 1999;94:2955–62.
53. Rösen-Wolff A, Soldan W, Heyne K, et al. Increased susceptibility of a carrier of X-linked chronic granulomatous disease (CGD) to Aspergillus fumigatus infection associated with age-related skewing of lyonization. Ann Hematol 2001;80:113–5.
54. Brandrup F, Koch C, Petri M, et al. Discoid lupus erythematosus-like lesions and stomatitis in female carriers of X-linked chronic granulomatous disease. Br J Dermatol 1981;104:495–505.
55. Kragballe K, Borregaard N, Brandrup F, et al. Relation of monocyte and neutro-phil oxidative metabolism to skin and oral lesions in carriers of chronic granulo-matous disease. Clin Exp Immunol 1981;43:390–8.
56. Rupec RA, Petropoulou T, Belohradsky BH, et al. Lupus erythematosus tumidus and chronic discoid lupus erythematosus in carriers of X-linked chronic granulo-matous disease. Eur J Dermatol 2000;10:184–9.
57. Margolis DM, Melnick DA, Alling DW, et al. Trimethoprim-sulfamethoxazole prophylaxis in the management of chronic granulomatous disease. J Infect Dis 1990;162:723–6.
58. International Chronic Granulomatous Disease Cooperative Study Group. A controlled trial of interferon gamma to prevent infection in chronic granuloma-tous disease. N Engl J Med 1991;324:509–16.
59. Rex JH, Bennett JE, Gallin JI, et al. In vivo interferon-gamma therapy augments the in vitro ability of chronic granulomatous disease neutrophils to damage Asper-gillus hyphae. J Infect Dis 1991;163:849–52.
60. Jackson SH, Miller GF, Segal BH, et al. IFN-gamma is effective in reducing infec-tions in the mouse model of chronic granulomatous disease (CGD). J Interferon Cytokine Res 2001;21:567–73.
61. Seger RA, Gungor T, Belohradsky BH, et al. Treatment of chronic granulomatous disease with myeloablative conditioning and an unmodified hemopoietic allograft: a survey of the European experience, 1985–2000. Blood 2002;100: 4344–50.
62. Kang EM, Marciano BE, DeRavin S, et al. Chronic granulomatous disease: over-view and hematopoietic stem cell transplantation. J Allergy Clin Immunol 2011; 127(6):1319–26.
63. Ozsahin H, von Planta M, Muller I, et al. Successful treatment of invasive aspergillosis in chronic granulomatous disease by bone marrow transplantation, granulocyte colony-stimulating factor-mobilized granulocytes, and liposomal amphotericin-B. Blood 1998;92:2719–24.

64. Horwitz ME, Barrett AJ, Brown MR, et al. Treatment of chronic granulomatous disease with nonmyeloablative conditioning and T-cell-depleted hematopoietic allograft. N Engl J Med 2001;344:881–8.
65. Kang EM, Malech HL. Gene therapy for chronic granulomatous disease. Meth Enzymol 2012;507:125–54.
66. Kono H, Rusyn I, Yin M, et al. NADPH oxidase-derived free radicals are key oxidants in alcohol-induced liver disease. J Clin Invest 2000;106:867–72.
67. Rusyn I, Kadiiska MB, Dikalova A, et al. Phthalates rapidly increase production of reactive oxygen species in vivo: role of Kupffer cells. Mol Pharmacol 2001;59: 744–50.
68. Barry-Lane PA, Patterson C, van der Merwe M, et al. p47phox is required for atherosclerotic lesion progression in ApoE (-/-) mice. J Clin Invest 2001;108: 1513–22.
69. Walder CE, Green SP, Darbonne WC, et al. Ischemic stroke injury is reduced in mice lacking a functional NADPH oxidase. Stroke 1997;28:2252–8.
70. Kishida KT, Hoeffer CA, Hu D, et al. Synaptic plasticity deficits and mild memory impairments in mouse models of chronic granulomatous disease. Mol Cell Biol 2006;26:5908–20.
71. Pao M, Wiggs EA, Anastacio MM, et al. Cognitive function in patients with chronic granulomatous disease: a preliminary report. Psychosomatics 2004;45:230–4.

Leukocyte Adhesion Deficiencies

Edith van de Vijver, MSc[a,b], Timo K. van den Berg, PhD[b],
Taco W. Kuijpers, MD, PhD[a],*

KEYWORDS

- Inflammation • Leukocytes • Leukocyte adhesion deficiency • β integrins • LAD-I
- LAD-II • LAD-III • Kindlin-3

KEY POINTS

- During inflammation, leukocytes play a key role in maintaining tissue homeostasis by elimination of pathogens and removal of damaged tissue.
- Leukocytes migrate to the site of inflammation by crawling over and through the blood vessel wall, into the tissue.
- Leukocyte adhesion deficiencies (ie, LAD-I, -II, and LAD-I/variant, the latter also known as LAD-III) are caused by defects in the adhesion of leukocytes to the blood vessel wall, due to mutations in the genes encoding β2 integrin (*ITGB2*), a GDP-fucose transport protein (*SLC35C1*) and kindlin-3 (*FERMT3*), respectively.
- Patients experience recurrent nonpussing bacterial infections and neutrophilia, often preceded by delayed separation of the umbilical cord, and additional symptoms depending on the subtype.
- For LAD-I and LAD-III, the only curative treatment is hematopoietic stem cell transplantation. In case of LAD-II, oral fucose supplementation may invert the immune defect, but additional mental retardation is hardly improved.

INTRODUCTION
Leukocyte Recruitment and Extravasation

During inflammation, circulating leukocytes migrate to the site of infection following a gradient of chemotaxins in a process called *chemotaxis*.[1] Chemotaxins may be derived from either the infected tissue or local complement activation, or directly from the pathogens themselves, and diffuse within the tissue into the local vasculature.[2] These gradients of chemotaxins recruit the leukocytes in interplay with factors expressed locally on the luminal side of blood vessel endothelial cells. Neutrophils are short-living leukocytes that are recruited early in the inflammatory response.

Leukocytes following the chemotaxin gradient toward the site of infection must leave the bloodstream, in a process called *extravasation* (**Fig. 1**).[1,3] Extravasation is

[a] Emma Children's Hospital, Academic Medical Centre, University of Amsterdam, Amsterdam, The Netherlands; [b] Department of Blood Cell Research, Sanquin Research and Landsteiner Laboratory, Amsterdam, The Netherlands
* Corresponding author.
E-mail address: t.w.kuijpers@amc.uva.nl

Hematol Oncol Clin N Am 27 (2013) 101–116
http://dx.doi.org/10.1016/j.hoc.2012.10.001

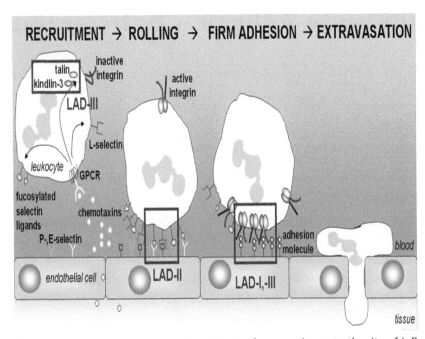

Fig. 1. Leukocyte recruitment and extravasation. Leukocytes migrate to the site of inflammation following a gradient of chemotaxins. The cells slow down because of transient interactions between selectins and their glycosylated ligands, which are defective in LAD-II. Next, stable adhesion by leukocyte integrins, absent in LAD-I, to ligands on the endothelium results in leukocyte arrest. Activation of blood cell integrins is decreased in LAD-III. Healthy neutrophils extravasate after firm adhesion.

a multistep process involving adhesion molecules, in which chemotaxins function as activating agents or (pro-) inflammatory mediators. The first step of extravasation consists of initial contact between endothelial cells and leukocytes marginated by the fluid flow of the blood. L-selectin (CD62L) on leukocytes plays a role herein, contacting several cell adhesion molecules on endothelial cells.[4] Within the local environment of an inflammatory tissue reaction, the endothelium begins to express the adhesion molecules P-selectin (CD62P) and later E-selectin (CD62E). The low-avidity interaction of these selectins with their fucosylated ligands on the opposite cells forces the leukocytes to slow down and start a rolling movement along the vessel wall (see **Fig. 1**).[4,5]

In contrast to the low-avidity binding of leukocytes to selectins, the final step of firm adhesion and subsequent migration depends on stable interaction between integrins on the leukocytes and their ligands on the endothelial cells.[1,6] Integrins are type 1 transmembrane glycoproteins that form heterodimers via noncovalent association of their α and β subunits, with sizes of 120 to 170 kDa and 90 to 130 kDa, respectively.[7] In mammals, 18 α and 8 β subunits form 24 known combinations, each of which can bind to a specific repertoire of cell-surface, extracellular matrix or soluble protein ligands. The β_2 integrin receptor subfamily is selectively expressed on leukocytes and comprises 4 different heterodimeric proteins, each of which contains a different α subunit: $\alpha_L\beta_2$ (LFA-1; CD11a/CD18), $\alpha_M\beta_2$ (CR3; CD11b/CD18), $\alpha_x\beta_2$ (gp150,95; CD11c/CD18); and $\alpha_D\beta_2$ (CD11d/CD18), the latter only being expressed on macrophages. The β_2 integrins bind to adhesion molecules on endothelial cells (intercellular adhesion molecule [ICAM]-1 and ICAM-2) and to several complement factors. The main β_2 integrin on neutrophils is CR3.[8]

Slowly rolling leukocytes are able to recognize concentration differences in a gradient of chemotaxins and to direct their movement toward the source of these agents. Although the details of this process remain unknown, the gradient most likely causes a difference in the number of ligand-bound chemotaxin receptors on either side of the cell, thereby inducing the cytoskeletal rearrangements needed for movement.[9] Because adhesion molecules such as the β_2 integrins are essential for the connections with the tissue cells or the extracellular matrix proteins, these connections must be formed at the front of the moving leukocytes and broken at the rear end.[10,11] Moreover, for continued sensing of the chemotaxin gradient, the chemotaxins must dissociate from their respective receptors for repeated use. This dissociation occurs through internalization of the ligand–receptor complex, intracellular disruption of the connection, and transport of the free receptor to the front of the cell, followed by reappearance of the free receptor on the leukocyte surface. Within the infected tissue, the chemotaxin gradient persists and leukocyte migration is maintained.

Integrin Activation

The ligand specificity of integrins is determined by their large extracellular ligand-binding head domain, which is composed of several domains of the α and β subunits.[12] The head domain is attached to the membrane via 2 flexible legs (1 from each subunit), which terminate intracellularly as short cytoplasmic tails. This domain architecture of integrins underlies their ability to transduce bidirectional signals across the plasma membrane: "inside-out" and "outside-in" (**Fig. 2**).[7,13] Leukocyte activation (eg, resulting from chemokine binding to chemokine receptors, ligand binding to selectins, or

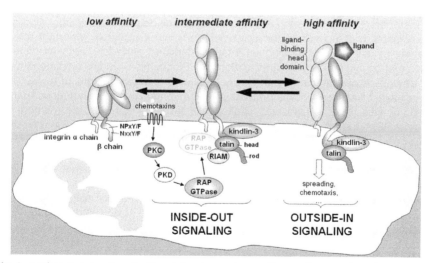

Fig. 2. Leukocyte integrin activation. Integrins are heterodimers of an α and a β chain, consisting of an extracellular ligand-binding head, a transmembrane domain, and 2 short cytoplasmic tails. Leukocyte activation (eg, by chemotaxin binding) causes inside-out signaling. This intracellular signaling, in which talin and kindlin play an important role, induces a conformational change resulting in increased ligand affinity. Subsequent ligand binding initiates downstream outside-in signaling, in which talin and kindlin may participate again, leading to reversible shuttling to a high-affinity conformation. Together with integrin clustering, this high-affinity conformation allows adhesion-mediated processes, such as cell spreading and chemotaxis.

antigen binding to the T-cell receptor) and subsequent intracellular signaling induces conformational changes in the extracellular regions of the β_2 integrins, leading to an enhanced affinity for their ligands (inside-out signaling). In addition, integrins cluster in larger complexes, which increases their ligand avidity. Binding to extracellular ligands leads to further conformational changes of the β_2 integrins, resulting in high ligand affinity, subsequent recruitment of cytosolic proteins, and the initiation of downstream signaling cascades that regulate cell spreading and alter gene expression, cell proliferation, differentiation, and apoptosis (outside-in signaling).[13]

The common activator of most, if not all, integrins is talin, a large cytoskeletal protein that acts as an allosteric activator of integrins by inducing their ligand-binding affinity.[12,14] The head domain of talin contains a FERM (4.1 protein, ezrin, radixin, moesin) domain, consisting of 3 subdomains: F1, F2, and F3. The F3 subdomain contains a phosphotyrosine-binding (PTB)–like domain that binds to the NPxY/F motif found in the membrane-proximal cytoplasmic region of several β integrins.[15] The head domain is connected to a long cytoplasmic rod that can interact with the cytoskeleton, allowing talin to contribute substantially to adhesion and motility via outside-in signaling cascades.[13]

Although binding of talin seems to be the final step in integrin activation, the activity of talin itself may be regulated by a variety of cell type–specific signaling pathways.[13,16] A study on chinese hamster ovary (CHO) cells expressing platelet integrins αIIb and $\beta3$ proposed that PKCα, activated by phorbol ester phorbol-12-myristate-acetate (PMA) or T-cell receptor stimulation, phosphorylates PKD1, which associates with a small GTPase from the Rap or Ras family that in turn activates the integrin upon formation of an activation complex with its effector protein Rap1-GTP-interacting adaptor molecule (RIAM) and talin.[17]

More recently, kindlin proteins have arisen as key players in integrin activation. Kindlins comprise a family of integrin-binding proteins.[18,19] In man, the family consists of 3 members: kindlin-1, -2, and -3, which share a high degree of homology. Kindlin-3 is expressed in all hematopoietic cell types, in which it plays an important role in a variety of functions depending on integrin-mediated adhesion, such as platelet clot formation and leukocyte extravasation.[20,21] Biochemical studies have confirmed that all kindlins directly bind synthetically generated cytoplasmic tails of β_1, β_2, and β_3 integrins.[19] Because kindlins possess a FERM domain that is homologous to that of talin, it was hypothesized that kindlins, like talin, interact with the membrane-proximal NPxY/F motif in the cytoplasmic tail of β integrins. However, recent studies have shown that the kindlin-binding site of β integrins is distinct from the talin-binding site, ie, at a membrane-distal NxxY/F motif in the cytoplasmic integrin tail.[22] Biochemical studies with mutants of kindlin-2 have shown that the PTB domain in F3 is, similarly to talin, essential for integrin binding, in addition to the *N*-terminus of the protein being required for interaction with β_3.[22] Kindlins are essential for inside-out integrin activation, and recent reports indicate an additional role in downstream outside-in cascades.[13]

Leukocyte Adhesion Deficiency

Leukocyte adhesion deficiencies (ie, LADs I, II, and III, the latter also known as LAD-1/variant) are immunodeficiencies caused by defects in the adhesion of leukocytes (especially neutrophils) to the blood vessel wall.[23,24] As a result, patients with any LAD subtype experience severe bacterial infections and neutrophilia, often preceded by delayed separation of the umbilical cord (**Table 1**). LAD-II is characterized by additional developmental problems, whereas in LAD-III, the immune defects are supplemented by a Glanzmann thrombasthenia-like bleeding tendency.

Table 1
Characteristics of LAD-I, -II, and -III

	LAD-I	LAD-II	LAD-III
Physical examination			
Recurrent nonpurulent bacterial and fungal infections	++ (skin & mucosal, gingivitis, periodontitis; necrotizing)	+ (decreasing during childhood; periodontitis)	+ (all have bacterial, some have fungal)
Delayed separation of umbilical cord, wound healing defect	+ (common omphalitis)	–	+ (some omphalitis)
Dysmorphism	–	+ (growth retardation, short stature, coarse face)	–
Neural abnormalities	–	+ (mental retardation, autism, convulsions, cerebral atrophy)	–
Bleeding tendency	–	–	+
Imaging and additional testing			
Genetic defect	+ (*ITGB2*)	+ (*SLC35C1*)	+ (*FERMT3*)
Leukocytosis	+ (20.10^6 up to 140.10^6/mL)	+ (up to 150.10^6/mL during infections)	+ (20.10^6 up to 70.10^6/mL, of which 30%–90% are neutrophils)
Erythrocytosis	–	–	Hb, 6–9/12–14
Thrombocytosis	–	–	Plt, 20–320 (avg, 140)
Expression of integrins (CD18, CD11b)	1%–30%, or present but dysfunctional	+	+
Expression of fucosylated glycoconjugates	+	– (sLeX, LeX, H-antigen, N-glycans)	+
Neutrophil defects	+ (firm adhesion, chemotaxis)	+ (rolling)	+ (firm adhesion, chemotaxis, spreading)
Platelet defects	–	–	+ (aggregation)
Therapeutic options			
Antibiotics	+	+	+ (also prophylactic)
HSCT	+ (severe vs moderate)	?	+
Fucose supplementation	–	+	–
Granulocyte transfusion	+ (potential benefit established)		+ (potential benefit established)
Thrombocyte transfusion	–	–	++/– (varies per patient)
Survival without HSCT	Severe form: low Moderate form: better	High	Low (10%–20%) often prior siblings diseased

Abbreviations: Avg, average; Hb, hemoglobin; HSCT, hematopoietic stem cell transplantation; Plt, platelets; sLeX, sialyl Lewis X; LeX, Lewis X.

LAD-I

LAD-I (OMIM #116920) is an autosomal recessive disorder caused by decreased expression or functioning of CD18, the β subunit of the leukocyte β₂ integrins.[25] LAD-I was first described in the early 1980s, and since then several hundred patients have been reported.[26] Mutations are found in *ITGB2* (integrin β₂, CD18), the gene located at 21q22.3 (OMIM *600065) that encodes the β₂ integrin. So far, 86 different mutations have been reported.[27] Usually, this leads to the absence or decreased expression of the β₂ integrins on the leukocyte surface, but sometimes a normal expression of nonfunctional β₂ integrins is found. Decreased expression of the common β₂ subunit leads to a similar decrease in the expression of all 4 α subunits on the leukocyte surface.

Physical Examination

LAD-I manifests through recurrent, life-threatening bacterial and fungal infections, primarily localized to skin and mucosal surfaces.[25,28] Infections are usually apparent from birth onward, together with severe septicemia in some patients, and a common presenting feature is omphalitis with delayed separation of the umbilical cord (**Fig. 3**). Later patients develop nonpurulent necrotizing infections of the skin and mucous membranes, resulting in a high mortality rate at an early age. Absence of pus formation at the sites of infection is a hallmark, and the infections have a high tendency for recurrence; secondary bacteremias may also occur. Among patients who survive infancy, severe gingivitis and chronic periodontitis are major features.[28,29] Fungal infections may present in individual cases.

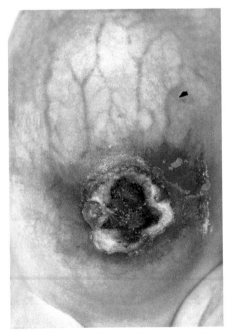

Fig. 3. Tissue necrosis after removal of the umbilical stump. Patients with LAD-I and -III commonly present with delayed separation of the umbilical cord, often followed by omphalitis, resulting in tissue necrosis in some cases.

Imaging and Additional Testing

Patients with LAD-I exhibit mild to moderate leukocytosis, especially granulocytosis, with neutrophil counts reaching levels greater than 100,000/mL during acute infection.[29] Because of the lack of adhesive capacity, only few, if any, leukocytes are present at the sites of infection, which are most often caused by *Staphylococcus aureus,* gram-negative enteric organisms, or fungi.

Definitive diagnosis of LAD-I is based on genetic analysis, revealing mutations in *ITGB2.* Flow cytometry with antibodies to detect CD18 allows discrimination of 2 forms of LAD-I: a severe form with less than 2% CD18 expression and a moderate form with 2% to 30% of expression.[30] A rare third group with severe symptoms exhibits normal expression of a functionally defective mutant protein. The severity of clinical presentation and complications in LAD-I correlates with the percentage of leukocytes showing normal CR3 cell surface expression and/or degree of molecule deficiency. Patients with severe LAD-I exhibit earlier, more frequent, and more serious episodes of infection, often leading to death in infancy, whereas patients with a moderate to mild phenotype experience fewer serious infectious episodes and commonly survive into adulthood.

Extensive in vitro studies on neutrophil functions have shown a marked defect in random migration and chemotaxis to various chemoattractants. Adhesion to and transmigration across endothelial cell layers were found to be severely impaired. Neutrophils fail to mobilize to skin sites in the in vivo Rebuck skin window test.[31]

Therapeutic Options

Antibiotics are commonly used to prevent and specifically treat acute or recurrent infections, and patients affected with the moderate form may survive to adulthood solely with antibiotics. As a curative treatment, hematopoietic stem cell transplantation (HSCT) is the only approach, and is most often the preferred treatment for patients with the severe form of LAD-I.[29,32]

Both reduced-intensity and myeloablative conditioning regimens are currently being used in HSCT of patients with LAD-I. With myeloablative conditioning, more complete depletion of host marrow can be achieved, thereby decreasing the possibility of mixed chimerism and the risk of rejection. However, pretransplant infections in immunodeficient patients lead to a high increase in mortality rates with this regimen, especially in patients with comorbid complications. Studies by Hamidieh and colleagues[32] show that use of the less toxic reduced-intensity conditioning (RIC) regimen is a more safe and feasible therapeutic approach to the treatment of patients with LAD-I. Recipients of RIC transplant, including those with either full or mixed chimerism, had a long-term survival rate with no manifestation of LAD-I symptoms.

Moreover, granulocyte transfusions have been reported to be a successful supplementation to LAD-I treatment. A patient who had an ecthyma gangrenosum lesion for 18 months, despite treatment with targeted antibiotics and antifungal therapy, was cured through massive granulocyte transfusions in association with granulocyte colony-stimulating factor (G-CSF).[33] Overall, the role of granulocyte transfusion in acute infectious episodes is debatable because of the associated side effects.

More recently, gene therapy has arisen as a potential treatment. Although gene therapy has been unsuccessful in humans with LAD-I, a study using foamy virus vectors in a canine leukocyte adhesion deficiency model was promising.[34,35]

Clinical Outcomes

The moderate form of LAD-I can often be controlled with prompt use of antibiotics during acute infectious episodes and, sometimes, prophylactic antibiotics. For patients with severe LAD-I, transplantation is commonly required at an early age. A multicenter study involving 36 patients showed an overall survival rate of 75%, with the best results from HLA-matched stem cell donors.[29]

Complications and Concerns

Frequent use of antibiotics may result in resistance of the bacteria. HSCT can be unsuccessful, especially in case of an incompletely matched donor.[29,32] Survival of HSCT treatment is lower than average for immunocompromised patients because of the risk of pretransplant infections. Although granulocyte transfusions have been added to treatment in some cases, the side effects may induce additional risks.[33]

LAD-II

The rare LAD-II syndrome was first reported in 1992 in 2 unrelated Arab Israeli boys, and to date fewer than 10 patients have been reported, with most from the Middle East.[36,37] Patients with LAD-II (OMIM #266265) have a defect in the fucosylation of various cell-surface glycoproteins, some of which function as selectin ligands, such as sialyl Lewis X carbohydrate groups (sLeX, CD15a).[38,39] As a result, a disturbance occurs in the initial rolling of leukocytes over the endothelial vessel wall in areas of inflammation, which is mediated by reversible contact between L-selectins on the leukocytes and E- or P-selectins on the endothelial cells, with their respective sialated fucosyl ligands on the opposite cells. Without rolling, the leukocytes cannot slow down and stably adhere, and in this way LAD-II leads to decreased leukocyte extravasation and recruitment to the site of infection. Fucosylation is also important for several unrelated functions, and as a result patients with LAD-II present with additional symptoms, including mental and growth retardation.[38,39]

The molecular defect in LAD-II has been identified as a deficiency in a Golgi GDP-fucose transport protein (GFTP).[40,41] This protein is encoded by *SLC35C1* (solute carrier family 35 member C1) or *FUCT1* (GDP-fucose transporter 1) at 11p11.2 (OMIM *605881), in which 7 different mutations have been reported so far.[27] Because the genetic cause reveals that the defect involves glycosylation, LAD-II has been categorized as one of the congenital disorders of glycosylation (CDGs), and has been reclassified as CDG-IIc.[40]

Physical Examination

The clinical course of LAD-II with respect to infectious complications is a milder one than LAD-I, in accordance with lower leukocyte counts. Although rolling is defective in patients with LAD-II, the adhesion and transmigration via β_2 integrin is intact, thereby permitting apparently some neutrophil mobilization to sites of inflammation and allowing some level of neutrophil defense in tissues.[36,42] In addition, the mechanisms of β_2 integrin activation are still intact.[30,36] Although recurrent bacterial infections occur in almost all patients, they are often not severe and do not result in overt wound healing defects or necrotic lesions as in LAD-I. Most infections occur in the first years of life, although periodontitis has been reported at a later age.[38]

However, patients with LAD-II present with other abnormal features, such as growth retardation (short stature), mental retardation, and a coarse face (**Fig. 4**).[38,39] Patients are born at term, with no apparent dysmorphism, but severely impaired postnatal weight gain and microcephaly are reported in most patients. In some families, intrauterine growth retardation was sufficient to screen for LAD-II prenatally. In addition, convulsions, cerebral atrophy, and autistic features were reported for more than half of the patients.[38] One patient had coronal craniosynostosis.[42]

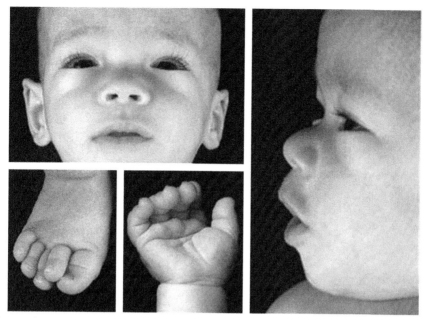

Fig. 4. Clinical stigmata in patients with LAD-II. Defective fucosylation results in growth retardation and a coarse face. Long eyelashes, a broad and depressed nasal bridge, a simian crease, and dorsally positioned second toes are the clinical stigmata of a patient with LAD-II. (*From* Marquardt T, Brune T, Luhn K, et al. Leukocyte adhesion deficiency II syndrome, a generalized defect in fucose metabolism. J Pediatr 1999;134(6):681–8; with permission.)

The early and late features of LAD-II, namely moderate immunodeficiency accompanied by neutrophilia in the first few years of life and severe mental retardation and short stature in childhood, are also prominent features of other CDGs.

Imaging and Additional Testing

The biochemical hallmark of LAD-II is a lack of expression of fucosylated glycoconjugates, such as the Lewis antigens Lewis X (LeX) and sialyl Lewis X (sLeX) on leukocyte proteins, α1,6-core fucosylated N-glycans on fibroblast proteins, and blood group antigen H on erythrocytes, the latter known as the rare *Bombay blood group* phenotype.[38,43] Expression of CR3 on LAD-II neutrophils is normal.[44,45]

Neutrophil values range from 6000 to greater than 50,000/mL in the absence of infection and up to 30,000 to 150,000/mL during infectious episodes.[36,46] With intravital microscopy, LAD-II neutrophils were found to roll poorly, only 5%, whereas the rolling fraction of control and LAD-I neutrophils is around 30%.[38] The neutrophil counts remain high during childhood and then decline at adolescence; this finding might be explained by an improvement in adaptive immunity with age, providing better defense against infections and reducing the stimuli for neutrophilia.[38]

Final proof of LAD-II arises from genetic analysis of the *SLC35C1* gene. The mutation seems to determine the severity of LAD-II: although GFTP is improperly located in the endoplasmic reticulum in some patients, it is directed to the Golgi but still dysfunctional in others, the latter correlated with a milder immunologic phenotype.[38]

Therapeutic Options and Clinical Outcome

Infections are commonly treated with antibiotics. In addition, high-dose oral supplementation with fucose had strong beneficial effects in some patients.[39,43,47] During 9 months of treatment with fucose in the first patients, infections and fever disappeared, elevated neutrophil counts returned to normal, and even psychomotor capabilities improved in one of the patients. However, fucose supplementation is not successful in all patients, because treatment of 2 Israeli Arab patients did not exhibit a similar beneficial response.[48] In addition, for one of the patients, treatment led to an autoimmune response against refucosylated antigens.[47] On discontinuation of therapy, selectin ligands were lost and neutrophil counts increased again within 7 days.[49]

Complications and Concerns

The metabolic pathways causing the severe psychomotor and growth retardation are still unclear. Oral fucose supplementation may cure immunologic symptoms in some cases, but developmental delay is hardly improving.[39]

LAD-III, LAD-1/v

LAD-III, also known as LAD-1/variant, was first described in 1997 by the authors' group and has now been identified in approximately 20 families worldwide.[24,27,50,52-59] In addition to recurrent nonpurulent infections, patients with LAD-III exhibit a severe Glanzmann thrombasthenia–like bleeding disorder.[24,51] Families have often lost newborns within weeks after birth, previous to the diagnosis of the reported patients, demonstrating the high mortality rate of these patients. The bleeding disorder originates from a platelet defect, indicating that the signaling defect also affects the β_3 integrin fibrinogen receptor $\alpha IIb\beta 3$ on blood platelets.

Since 2010, the molecular defect of this variant form of LAD (OMIM #612840) has been assigned to mutations in *FERMT3* (fermitin family homolog 3) at 11q13.1 (OMIM *607901).[27] *FERMT3* encodes kindlin-3, a protein involved in inside-out signaling to all blood cell–expressed β integrins (β_1, β_2, and β_3).[44,60] So far, 11 different mutations in *FERMT3* have been reported.[27,50,55]

A discussion has occurred in the literature about the importance of a genetic variation in the gene encoding CalDAG-GEF1 (a guanine nucleotide exchange factor for Rap1, involved in integrin activation) in some patients with LAD-III, in addition to mutations in *FERMT3* found in these patients.[52,56,61] However, because the functional defect in these patients can only be corrected through reconstitution with kindlin-3 and not reconstitution with CalDAG-GEF1, this variation in CalDAG-GEF1 is of no importance for the functional defect in patients with LAD-III.[59] Experiments with kindlin-3 knockout mice by Moser and colleagues[20,62] led to the original hypothesis of kindlin-3 deficiency in LAD-III, confirmed as indicated by the description of various mutations, and have subsequently been used as a tool to delve into LAD-III pathology.

Physical Examination

Patients with LAD-III experience severe recurrent nonpurulent infections, often preceded by delayed umbilical cord detachment with or without omphalitis, and leukocytosis, as is seen in patients with LAD-I.[23] In addition, patients with LAD-III are affected by a bleeding tendency, similar or more severe than that exhibited by patients with Glanzmann thrombasthenia.[51]

Some patients experiencing LAD-III may also present with an osteopetrosis-like bone defect in addition to the increased bleeding tendency and recurrent infections.[53,63] A prominent osteopetrosic phenotype was also observed in the kindlin-3 knockout mice. The cause of this osteopetrosis might lie within the osteoclasts, which represent macrophage-like hematopoietic cells critical for bone resorption. Bone resorption requires the formation of a so-called sealing zone that depends on αvβ3 integrin–mediated adhesion to the bone, thereby explaining the skeletal defect.[60] However, the prevalence and manifestations of osteopetrosis differ largely among patients with LAD-III, because unaffected bone formation is also found (**Fig. 5**). The reason for this heterogeneity has remained unclear.

Imaging and Additional Testing

Similar to LAD-I and -II, LAD-III should be confirmed through genetic analysis, which will reveal mutations in *FERMT3*. Expression of integrins on neutrophils and platelets (ie, αIIβ1, αIIbβ3) is normal or slightly increased, and integrin activation can be induced by artificial stimulation with monoclonal antibodies or cations.[44] Based on the persistent leukocytosis, juvenile myelomonocytic leukemia (JMML) was suspected in many of the patients.[64] However, the increased sensitivity of bone marrow or blood cells to granulocyte-macrophage colony-stimulating factor, as the hallmark for JMML, is negative in LAD-III.

Many tests have been performed on LAD-III neutrophils. One example of an assay to discriminate between LAD-I and LAD-III neutrophils is the NADPH oxidase screening test with unopsonized zymosan (UZ), as described by the authors' group.[64] UZ is used to induce uptake and NADPH oxidase activity in purified neutrophils based on the requirement for kindlin-3–dependent CR3 activation before uptake of the zymosan. The response is absent in both types of LAD, but activation and subsequent zymosan uptake can be induced by high Mg^{2+} concentrations only in case of LAD-III, proving that CR3, once in its active conformation, is functional in these patients. Similarly,

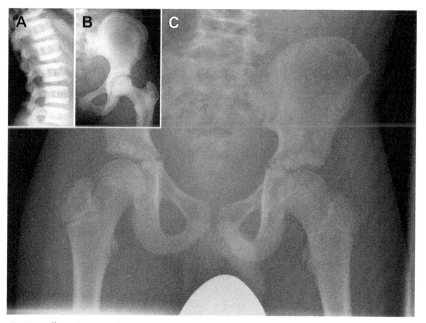

Fig. 5. Not all patients with LAD-III show osteopetrosis. Vertebrae and hip joint of an osteopetrotic patient (*A, B*) compared with the lumbar vertebrae and pelvis of a patient who is kindlin-3–deficient without osteopetrosis (*C*).

neutrophil adhesion to CR3 ligands is absent in response to several chemoattractants, but can be induced with Mn^{2+} on artificial integrin activation.

In addition to the recurrent infections, patients with LAD-III experience a bleeding tendency, which has been reported to be more severe than in Glanzmann thrombasthenia. With a novel flow cytometric aggregation assay, both syndromes can be discriminated based on formation of small aggregates.[65] Platelets from patients with Glanzmann thrombasthenia are still capable of forming small aggregates on collagen stimulation, whereas platelets from patients with LAD-III are not. These aggregates require functional GPIa/IIa (integrin $\alpha2\beta1$), thus explaining the clinically more severe bleeding manifestations in patients with LAD-III, in whom all platelet integrins are functionally defective.

Erythrocytes of kindlin-3-/- mice are abnormally shaped, with striking protrusions and invaginations. The cells have altered expression levels of cytoskeletal proteins, and the mice are severely anemic. In humans with LAD-III, the authors and others have seen less prominent alterations of the erythrocyte population, including dacrocytes (teardrop–shaped) and elliptocytes (**Fig. 6**).[55] Altered levels of cytoskeletal proteins have not been reported.

Splenomegaly or hepatosplenomegaly has been observed in almost all patients, in some only later during infancy, which may result from extramedullary hematopoiesis. Besides expression in hematopoietic cells, low kindlin-3 levels also have been reported in endothelial cells, although the biologic significance is unclear.[66]

Therapeutic Options

Patients with LAD-III need prophylactic antibiotics and repeated blood transfusions, but the only curative therapy is HSCT. For untransplanted patients, the urge for transfusion differs per patient and can increase to more than 20 and 50 transfusions per year for erythrocytes and platelets, respectively.[64] In addition, granulocyte transfusions have been used in at least 1 patient and are believed to increase pathogen clearance.[64]

Clinical Outcomes

The survival of untransplanted patients with LAD-III is low, and the high mortality is further demonstrated by the incidence of deceased siblings who were not diagnosed

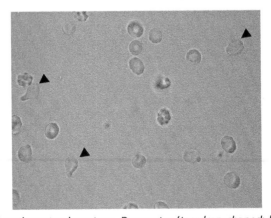

Fig. 6. Abnormal erythrocyte phenotype. Dacrocytes (teardrop–shaped; left 2 arrowheads) and elliptocytes (right arrowhead) characterize the erythrocyte population of LAD III, although the phenotype is less severe than in kindlin-3-/- mice.

but experienced similar symptoms. Fewer than 4 patients have so far survived childhood without HSCT, and the oldest reported patient has reached the age of 20 years, although the need for platelet transfusions has increased to 1 to 2 transfusions per week. On successful HSCT, patients may continue live without further symptoms.

Complications and Concerns

Although the success rate for HSCT has improved over the past years, pretransplant infections and the bleeding disorder often cause major complications in the treatment of patients with LAD-III. In addition, osteopetrosis may complicate the conditioning regimen.[67]

ACKNOWLEDGMENTS

The authors gratefully acknowledge Prof. Dirk Roos for critically reading the manuscript.

REFERENCES

1. Ley K, Laudanna C, Cybulsky MI, et al. Getting to the site of inflammation: the leukocyte adhesion cascade updated. Nat Rev Immunol 2007;7(9):678–89.
2. Murdoch C, Finn A. Chemokine receptors and their role in inflammation and infectious diseases. Blood 2000;95(10):3032–43.
3. Zimmerman GA, Prescott SM, McIntyre TM. Endothelial cell interactions with granulocytes: tethering and signaling molecules. Immunol Today 1992;13(3): 93–100.
4. Zarbock A, Ley K, McEver RP, et al. Leukocyte ligands for endothelial selectins: specialized glycoconjugates that mediate rolling and signaling under flow. Blood 2011;118(26):6743–51.
5. Kansas GS. Selectins and their ligands: current concepts and controversies. Blood 1996;88(9):3259–87.
6. Barreiro O, Sanchez-Madrid F. Molecular basis of leukocyte-endothelium interactions during the inflammatory response. Rev Esp Cardiol 2009;62(5):552–62.
7. Hynes RO. Integrins: bidirectional, allosteric signaling machines. Cell 2002; 110(6):673–87.
8. Schymeinsky J, Mocsai A, Walzog B. Neutrophil activation via beta2 integrins (CD11/CD18): molecular mechanisms and clinical implications. Thromb Haemost 2007;98(2):262–73.
9. Delon I, Brown NH. Integrins and the actin cytoskeleton. Curr Opin Cell Biol 2007; 19(1):43–50.
10. Kuijpers TW, Hakkert BC, Hart MH, et al. Neutrophil migration across monolayers of cytokine-prestimulated endothelial cells: a role for platelet-activating factor and IL-8. J Cell Biol 1992;117(3):565–72.
11. Springer TA. Traffic signals for lymphocyte recirculation and leukocyte emigration: the multistep paradigm. Cell 1994;76(2):301–14.
12. Calderwood DA, Zent R, Grant R, et al. The Talin head domain binds to integrin beta subunit cytoplasmic tails and regulates integrin activation. J Biol Chem 1999;274(40):28071–4.
13. Hogg N, Patzak I, Willenbrock F. The insider's guide to leukocyte integrin signalling and function. Nat Rev Immunol 2011;11(6):416–26.
14. Lim J, Wiedemann A, Tzircotis G, et al. An essential role for talin during alpha(M) beta(2)-mediated phagocytosis. Mol Biol Cell 2007;18(3):976–85.

15. Garcia-Alvarez B, de Pereda JM, Calderwood DA, et al. Structural determinants of integrin recognition by talin. Mol Cell 2003;11(1):49–58.
16. Shattil SJ, Kim C, Ginsberg MH. The final steps of integrin activation: the end game. Nat Rev Mol Cell Biol 2010;11(4):288–300.
17. Han J, Lim CJ, Watanabe N, et al. Reconstructing and deconstructing agonist-induced activation of integrin alphaIIbbeta3. Curr Biol 2006;16(18):1796–806.
18. Kahner BN, Kato H, Banno A, et al. Kindlins, integrin activation and the regulation of talin recruitment to alphaIIbbeta3. PLoS One 2012;7(3):e34056.
19. Malinin NL, Plow EF, Byzova TV. Kindlins in FERM adhesion. Blood 2010;115(20): 4011–7.
20. Moser M, Bauer M, Schmid S, et al. Kindlin-3 is required for beta2 integrin-mediated leukocyte adhesion to endothelial cells. Nat Med 2009;15(3):300–5.
21. Nieswandt B, Varga-Szabo D, Elvers M. Integrins in platelet activation. J Thromb Haemost 2009;7(Suppl):1206–9.
22. Harburger DS, Bouaouina M, Calderwood DA. Kindlin-1 and -2 directly bind the C-terminal region of beta integrin cytoplasmic tails and exert integrin-specific activation effects. J Biol Chem 2009;284(17):11485–97.
23. Etzioni A. Defects in the leukocyte adhesion cascade. Clin Rev Allergy Immunol 2010;38(1):54–60.
24. Kuijpers TW, Van Lier RA, Hamann D, et al. Leukocyte adhesion deficiency type 1 (LAD-1)/variant. A novel immunodeficiency syndrome characterized by dysfunctional beta2 integrins. J Clin Invest 1997;100(7):1725–33.
25. Hanna S, Etzioni A. Leukocyte adhesion deficiencies. Ann N Y Acad Sci 2012; 1250:50–5.
26. Crowley CA, Curnutte JT, Rosin RE, et al. An inherited abnormality of neutrophil adhesion. Its genetic transmission and its association with a missing protein. N Engl J Med 1980;302(21):1163–8.
27. van de Vijver E, Maddalena A, Sanal O, et al. Hematologically important mutations: leukocyte adhesion deficiency (first update). Blood Cells Mol Dis 2012;48(1):53–61.
28. Movahedi M, Entezari N, Pourpak Z, et al. Clinical and laboratory findings in Iranian patients with leukocyte adhesion deficiency (study of 15 cases). J Clin Immunol 2007;27(3):302–7.
29. Qasim W, Cavazzana-Calvo M, Davies EG, et al. Allogeneic hematopoietic stem-cell transplantation for leukocyte adhesion deficiency. Pediatrics 2009;123(3):836–40.
30. Fischer A, Lisowska-Grospierre B, Anderson DC, et al. Leukocyte adhesion deficiency: molecular basis and functional consequences. Immunodefic Rev 1988; 1(1):39–54.
31. von Andrian UH, Berger EM, Ramezani L, et al. In vivo behavior of neutrophils from two patients with distinct inherited leukocyte adhesion deficiency syndromes. J Clin Invest 1993;91(6):2893–7.
32. Hamidieh AA, Pourpak Z, Hosseinzadeh M, et al. Reduced-intensity conditioning hematopoietic SCT for pediatric patients with LAD-1: clinical efficacy and importance of chimerism. Bone Marrow Transplant 2012;47(5):646–50.
33. Mellouli F, Ksouri H, Barbouche R, et al. Successful treatment of Fusarium solani ecthyma gangrenosum in a patient affected by leukocyte adhesion deficiency type 1 with granulocytes transfusions. BMC Dermatol 2010;10:10.
34. Bauer TR Jr, Allen JM, Hai M, et al. Successful treatment of canine leukocyte adhesion deficiency by foamy virus vectors. Nat Med 2008;14(1):93–7.
35. Hunter MJ, Zhao H, Tuschong LM, et al. Gene therapy for canine leukocyte adhesion deficiency with lentiviral vectors using the murine stem cell virus and human phosphoglycerate kinase promoters. Hum Gene Ther 2011;22(6):689–96.

36. Etzioni A, Frydman M, Pollack S, et al. Brief report: recurrent severe infections caused by a novel leukocyte adhesion deficiency. N Engl J Med 1992;327(25): 1789–92.
37. Marquardt T, Brune T, Luhn K, et al. Leukocyte adhesion deficiency II syndrome, a generalized defect in fucose metabolism. J Pediatr 1999;134(6):681–8.
38. Gazit Y, Mory A, Etzioni A, et al. Leukocyte adhesion deficiency type II: long-term follow-up and review of the literature. J Clin Immunol 2010;30(2):308–13.
39. Yakubenia S, Wild MK. Leukocyte adhesion deficiency II. Advances and open questions. FEBS J 2006;273(19):4390–8.
40. Lubke T, Marquardt T, Etzioni A, et al. Complementation cloning identifies CDG-IIc, a new type of congenital disorders of glycosylation, as a GDP-fucose transporter deficiency. Nat Genet 2001;28(1):73–6.
41. Luhn K, Wild MK, Eckhardt M, et al. The gene defective in leukocyte adhesion deficiency II encodes a putative GDP-fucose transporter. Nat Genet 2001;28(1):69–72.
42. Frydman M, Etzioni A, Eidlitz-Markus T, et al. Rambam-Hasharon syndrome of psychomotor retardation, short stature, defective neutrophil motility, and Bombay phenotype. Am J Med Genet 1992;44(3):297–302.
43. Marquardt T, Luhn K, Srikrishna G, et al. Correction of leukocyte adhesion deficiency type II with oral fucose. Blood 1999;94(12):3976–85.
44. McDowall A, Inwald D, Leitinger B, et al. A novel form of integrin dysfunction involving beta1, beta2, and beta3 integrins. J Clin Invest 2003;111(1):51–60.
45. Phillips ML, Schwartz BR, Etzioni A, et al. Neutrophil adhesion in leukocyte adhesion deficiency syndrome type 2. J Clin Invest 1995;96(6):2898–906.
46. Wild MK, Luhn K, Marquardt T, et al. Leukocyte adhesion deficiency II: therapy and genetic defect. Cells Tissues Organs 2002;172(3):161–73.
47. Hidalgo A, Ma S, Peired AJ, et al. Insights into leukocyte adhesion deficiency type 2 from a novel mutation in the GDP-fucose transporter gene. Blood 2003; 101(5):1705–12.
48. Etzioni A, Tonetti M. Fucose supplementation in leukocyte adhesion deficiency type II. Blood 2000;95(11):3641–3.
49. Luhn K, Marquardt T, Harms E, et al. Discontinuation of fucose therapy in LADII causes rapid loss of selectin ligands and rise of leukocyte counts. Blood 2001; 97(1):330–2.
50. Harris ES, Smith TL, Springett GM, et al. Leukocyte adhesion deficiency-I variant syndrome (LAD-Iv, LAD-III): molecular characterization of the defect in an index family. Am J Hematol 2012;87(3):311–3.
51. Jurk K, Schulz AS, Kehrel BE, et al. Novel integrin-dependent platelet malfunction in siblings with leukocyte adhesion deficiency-III (LAD-III) caused by a point mutation in FERMT3. Thromb Haemost 2010;103(5):1053–64.
52. Kuijpers TW, van de Vijver E, Weterman MA, et al. LAD-1/variant syndrome is caused by mutations in FERMT3. Blood 2009;113(19):4740–6.
53. Malinin NL, Zhang L, Choi J, et al. A point mutation in KINDLIN3 ablates activation of three integrin subfamilies in humans. Nat Med 2009;15(3):313–8.
54. McDowall A, Svensson L, Stanley P, et al. Two mutations in the KINDLIN3 gene of a new leukocyte adhesion deficiency III patient reveal distinct effects on leukocyte function in vitro. Blood 2010;115(23):4834–42.
55. Meller J, Malinin NL, Panigrahi S, et al. Novel aspects of Kindlin-3 function in humans based on a new case of leukocyte adhesion deficiency III (LAD-III). J Thromb Haemost 2012;10(7):1397–408.
56. Mory A, Feigelson SW, Yarali N, et al. Kindlin-3: a new gene involved in the pathogenesis of LAD-III. Blood 2008;112(6):2591.

57. Robert P, Canault M, Farnarier C, et al. A novel leukocyte adhesion deficiency III variant: kindlin-3 deficiency results in integrin- and nonintegrin-related defects in different steps of leukocyte adhesion. J Immunol 2011;186(9):5273–83.

58. Sabnis H, Kirpalani A, Horan J, et al. Leukocyte adhesion deficiency-III in an African-American patient. Pediatr Blood Cancer 2010;55(1):180–2.

59. Svensson L, Howarth K, McDowall A, et al. Leukocyte adhesion deficiency-III is caused by mutations in KINDLIN3 affecting integrin activation. Nat Med 2009; 15(3):306–12.

60. Schmidt S, Nakchbandi I, Ruppert R, et al. Kindlin-3-mediated signaling from multiple integrin classes is required for osteoclast-mediated bone resorption. J Cell Biol 2011;192(5):883–97.

61. Pasvolsky R, Feigelson SW, Kilic SS, et al. A LAD-III syndrome is associated with defective expression of the Rap-1 activator CalDAG-GEFI in lymphocytes, neutrophils, and platelets. J Exp Med 2007;204(7):1571–82.

62. Moser M, Nieswandt B, Ussar S, et al. Kindlin-3 is essential for integrin activation and platelet aggregation. Nat Med 2008;14(3):325–30.

63. Kilic SS, Etzioni A. The clinical spectrum of leukocyte adhesion deficiency (LAD) III due to defective CalDAG-GEF1. J Clin Immunol 2009;29(1):117–22.

64. Kuijpers TW, van Bruggen R, Kamerbeek N, et al. Natural history and early diagnosis of LAD-1/variant syndrome. Blood 2007;109(8):3529–37.

65. van de Vijver E, De Cuyper IM, Gerrits AJ, et al. Defects in Glanzmann thrombasthenia and LAD-III (LAD-1/v) syndrome: the role of integrin beta1 and beta3 in platelet adhesion to collagen. Blood 2012;119(2):583–6.

66. Bialkowska K, Ma YQ, Bledzka K, et al. The integrin co-activator Kindlin-3 is expressed and functional in a non-hematopoietic cell, the endothelial cell. J Biol Chem 2010;285(24):18640–9.

67. Elhasid R, Kilic SS, Ben-Arush M, et al. Prompt recovery of recipient hematopoiesis after two consecutive haploidentical peripheral blood SCTs in a child with leukocyte adhesion defect III syndrome. Bone Marrow Transplant 2010;45(2): 413–4.

Clinical and Molecular Pathophysiology of Shwachman–Diamond Syndrome: An Update

Kasiani C. Myers, MD[a],*, Stella M. Davies, MBBS, PhD, MRCP[b],
Akiko Shimamura, MD, PhD[c]

KEYWORDS

- Bone marrow failure • Shwachman–diamond syndrome • Ribosomes

KEY POINTS

- Many exciting advances in our understanding of SDS have occurred in the past few years.
- Our understanding of the natural history and spectrum of disease, diagnosis, and therapy remain limited.
- Ongoing basic and clinical investigations on larger numbers of patients are crucial to better tie together our evolving comprehension of molecular function and clinical manifestations of this multiorgan disease to affect the treatment of patients with this rare disorder.

INTRODUCTION

Shwachman–Diamond syndrome (SDS) is a rare autosomal recessive multisystem disorder characterized by congenital anomalies, exocrine pancreatic dysfunction, bone marrow failure, and predisposition to myelodysplasia (MDS) and leukemia, particularly acute myeloid leukemia (AML). In addition, growth, heart, liver, central nervous system, skeletal system, and the immune system may also be affected. The incidence of SDS is indirectly approximated at 1:77,000.[1] Around 90% of patients with SDS harbor mutations in the Shwachman-Bodian-Diamond syndrome (SBDS) gene located on chromosome 7q11. SBDS encodes a novel protein involved in ribosomal maturation and implicated in additional functions, such as cell proliferation and mitosis,[2] as well as in the stromal microenvironment.[3,4]

[a] Division of Bone Marrow Transplantation and Immune Deficiency, Cincinnati Children's Hospital Medical Center, University of Cincinnati, 3333 Burnet Avenue, MLC 7015, Cincinnati, OH 45229, USA; [b] Division of Bone Marrow Transplantation and Immune Deficiency, Cincinnati Children's Hospital Medical Center, University of Cincinnati, 3333 Burnet Avenue, Cincinnati, OH 45229, USA; [c] Department of Pediatric Hematology/Oncology, Fred Hutchinson Cancer Research Center, Seattle Children's Hospital, University of Washington, 4800 Sand Point Way NE, Seattle, WA 98105, USA
* Corresponding author.
E-mail address: kasiani.myers@cchmc.org

Hematol Oncol Clin N Am 27 (2013) 117–128
http://dx.doi.org/10.1016/j.hoc.2012.10.003
0889-8588/13/$ – see front matter © 2013 Elsevier Inc. All rights reserved.

Although the majority (90%)[5] of patients clinically diagnosed with SDS harbor mutations in the *SBDS* gene, phenotype varies widely between patients and even within the same individual over time, posing challenges for diagnosis and treatment. Owing to the rarity of this disorder, the natural history of SDS remains poorly defined and controlled clinical studies to direct therapy are lacking. Thus, current management is largely based on case series and consensus reports. Longitudinal clinical studies are needed to define the diagnostic criteria, phenotypic range, and molecular pathophysiology of SDS to identify risk factors for medical complications and guide therapeutic interventions.

This review highlights recent advances in the understanding of the clinical manifestations and molecular pathogenesis of SDS. The reader is referred to prior excellent reviews for a general overview of SDS.[6–8]

CLINICAL MANIFESTATIONS

Owing to the rarity of this syndrome, our understanding of the full spectrum of clinical disease in SDS remains incomplete. The current knowledge was summarized recently in an updated clinical consensus guideline.[6] The classical clinical scenario describing SDS includes exocrine pancreatic dysfunction and bone marrow failure (**Box 1**). Skeletal abnormalities may include metaphyseal dysplasia, flared ribs, thoracic dystrophies, and osteopenia.[9] Neurocognitive deficits have been described.[10] While the exocrine pancreatic dysfunction in SDS is well described, a distinctive abnormal hepatic phenotype in these patients has also been reported.[11] Progression and evolution of bone marrow disease remains a major source of morbidity and mortality in these patients.[12,13] Registries and clinically annotated biosample repositories for SDS are poised to expand our knowledge of this disease and its myriad of developmental effects through systematic and longitudinal studies leading to more disease-specific interventions.

HEMATOLOGIC MANIFESTATIONS

Patients with SDS are at risk for cytopenias secondary to marrow failure. Neutropenia is reported in 88% to 100% of patients and can be either intermittent or persistent, with variable severity. Anemia and thrombocytopenia have also been reported in most patients, although both are often intermittent or asymptomatic. Elevated hemoglobin F levels can also be seen in a subset of patients.[14,15] Severe aplastic anemia with trilineage cytopenias may also develop in a subset of patients. The French Severe Chronic Neutropenia Registry recently evaluated the hematologic complications in their cohort of 102 genetically diagnosed patients with SDS and found 41 patients (40%) with hematologic complications including transient severe cytopenias.[12] Of these patients, 21 (20.6%) presented with definitive persistent cytopenias (anemia with hemoglobin levels <7 g/dL or profound thrombocytopenia with platelets <20 g/L), in 9 of whom the condition was classified as malignant and in another 9 as nonmalignant, and in 3, the condition progressed from nonmalignant to malignant. Prognostic factors reported with severe cytopenias in this cohort included early age at diagnosis and hematologic parameters.

Reports of progression to MDS or AML in patients with SDS have varied. Previously, the Severe Chronic Neutropenia International Registry (SCNIR) had reported a rate of 1% per year of MDS or AML in patients with SDS, with an overall incidence of 8.1% in 37 patients with SDS in 10 years.[16,17] The French registry reported a rate of transformation to MDS or AML of 18.8% at 20 years and 36.1% at 30 years in a cohort of 55 patients with SDS.[18] Some of this discrepancy arises from differences in the definition of MDS. More recently, the Canadian Inherited Bone Marrow Failure Study (CIBMFS)

Box 1
Clinical and molecular diagnostic features of Shwachman–Diamond syndrome

Biallelic mutations in SBDS or clinical Shwachman–Diamond syndrome: one criteria from Category I and II

Category I

   Low levels of trypsinogen (age <3 years) *or* low pancreatic isoamylase levels (age >3 years)

   Low levels of fecal elastase

   Supportive features:

      Pancreatic lipomatosis

      Elevated 72-hour fecal fat excretion *and* absence of intestinal pathologic condition

Category II

   Hypoproductive cytopenias

      Neutropenia (absolute neutrophil count <1500)

      Anemia or idiopathic macrocytosis

      Thrombocytopenia (<150,000)

   Bone marrow examination with any of the following:

      Myelodysplasia

      Leukemia

      Myelodysplasia syndrome

      Hypocellularity for age

      Cytogenetic abnormalities

Supporting features

   First-degree or second-degree blood relative with Shwachman–Diamond syndrome

   Personal history of

      Congenital skeletal abnormalities consistent with chondrodysplasia or a congenital thoracic dystrophy

      Height 3% or less, of unclear cause

      Deficiency in 2 or more fat-soluble vitamins (A, 25-OHD, and E).

---

registry reported a cumulative transformation rate of 18% in 34 patients with SDS.[13] This result is in contrast to other recent reports from the NIH registry (17 patients) and the Israeli registry (3 patients) in which no patient developed MDS or AML.[19,20] Although it is difficult to draw conclusions from such small numbers of patients, this discrepancy may be partly due to the age of these cohorts. The median age of transformation for patients with SDS was 19.1 years in the French group and 20 years in the Canadian cohort, whereas the NIH and Israeli cohorts had median ages of 14 and 4 years, respectively, at the time of report.[13] Transformation rates reported by the SCNIR for patients with severe congenital neutropenia (SCN) are 11.8% at 10 years, whereas the rates for fanconi anemia (FA) and dyskeratosis congenita (DC) by the age of 50 years as reported by the NIH are 40% and 30%, respectively, for myelodysplasia (MDS), and 10% for both for AML.[17,19] The Diamond Blackfan Anemia Registry reports that patients with diamond blackfan anemia (DBA) are less likely to transform with cumulative incidence of AML of 5% by the age of 46 years, with incidence increasing only after the age of 40 years.[21] Together, these data suggest that the risk of malignant transformation in patients with SDS is significant, especially with respect to some of the other inherited marrow failure syndromes, but occurs with less frequency and longer latency than in patients with Fanconi anemia. Published reports of solid tumors in patients with SDS are rare thus far. There are only 2 cases in the literature, one of bilateral breast cancer[22] in a 30-year-old woman with SDS and another of dermatofibrosarcoma in a 20-year old-woman, which had been present and slowly growing for approximately 3 years at diagnosis.[23]

It has long been known that patients with SDS may develop characteristic cytogenetic clones in the absence of overt MDS or AML and that these abnormalities may persist over time without progression or malignant evolution. Recent reports suggest that a common cytogenetic abnormality seen in patients with SDS, del(20)(q11), is not associated with a high risk of malignant transformation.[24,25] Another characteristic cytogenetic anomaly in SDS that can come and go over years of time without progression to MDS/AML is isochromosome i(7)(q10).[26] Maserati and colleagues[25] reported on clonal changes in 22 new patients with SDS and 14 cases of follow-up of previously reported cases.[25] Of the 36 cases, 16 demonstrated clonal changes, all of which involved either chromosome 7 or 20. Chromosome 7 abnormalities included isochromosome [i(7)(q10) (n = 10)], [add(7)(p?) (n = 1)], and a long arm deletion [del(7)(q22q23) (n = 1)]. All 6 clones involving chromosome 20 abnormalities initially involved del(20)(q11); however, 2 evolved into subclones, which had acquired additional cytogenetic abnormalities. All 5 patients with del(20)(q11) demonstrated loss of the common MDR established in patients with MDS who did not have SDS. Over the course of the study (range of follow-up being between 1 month and 9 years), 8 patients had stable clones, 4 demonstrated increasing clonal involvement, and 1 had diminished clonal involvement, irrespective of the initial type or size of clonal abnormality. Despite these additional cytogenetic abnormalities and the loss of a region commonly deleted in MDS/AML, the only patient to progress to MDS or require bone marrow transplantation carried the add(7)(p?) abnormality, and no patient progressed to AML. In addition, the appearance of clonal abnormalities seemed to be age related, with increased frequency of clonal changes seen with increasing age.

Furthermore, Crescenzi and colleagues[24] evaluated the bone marrows of 2 patients with SDS and del(20)(q11) who had been followed up over a 6- to 7-year period without development of MDS/AML. In these patients, there was no acquisition of additional cytogenetic changes associated with MDS/AML despite increasing clonal population in 1 patient. By fluorescence in situ hybridization, del(20)(q11) was seen to be present in totipotent hematopoietic stem cells as well as downstream myeloid and lymphoid lineages, indicating preservation of the capacity to differentiate even in the face of this cytogenetic abnormality.

Historically, clinical observations have also demonstrated an increased frequency of infection beyond that attributable to simple neutropenia in patients with SDS. Sepsis is one of the most common fatal infections in SDS, often associated with neutropenia. However, patients with SDS also have susceptibility to recurrent bacterial, viral, and fungal infections.[27] Dror and colleagues[28] prospectively studied immune functions in this population. B-cell defects (less number of circulating B cell, low levels of IgG and IgG subclasses, and deficient antibody production) and T-cell defects (low $Cd3^+/CD4^+$ cell subpopulations and decreased T-lymphocyte proliferation) were described in most patients with SDS studied. Universally abnormal neutrophil chemotaxis was also reported as described previously.[29,30] However, in contrast to other neutrophil chemotaxis disorders, patients with SDS retain the ability to form purulent abscesses and empyema.[27]

GASTROINTESTINAL MANIFESTATIONS

Exocrine pancreatic dysfunction is a classic feature of SDS resulting from severe depletion of pancreatic acinar cells.[14,31] The majority (>90%) of patients with SDS are diagnosed with pancreatic dysfunction in the first year of life, often in the first 6 months. Clinical manifestations range widely from severe dysfunction with significant nutrient malabsorption, steatorrhea, and resultant failure to thrive, to completely asymptomatic. Despite these findings, clinical symptoms in many patients with SDS spontaneously improve with age for reasons that remain unclear. In as many as 50% of patients, pancreatic enzyme supplementation can be stopped by the age 4 years based on evidence of normal fat absorption, although enzyme secretion deficits remain.[32] A recent study of parotid acinar function in 16 patients with SDS compared with 13 healthy controls and 13 patients with cystic fibrosis or fibrosing pancreatitis found parotid acinar dysfunction.[33] Both serum pancreatic and parotid isoamylase levels were lower in patients with SDS than in healthy controls, whereas pancreatic isoamylase levels were lower in other disease controls than in normal controls. Secreted parotid amylase levels were also lower in patients with SDS than in healthy controls, whereas the levels in disease controls were comparable to those in normal controls. These findings suggest a more generalized defect in acinar cell function in patients with SDS. In addition, a recent study by Shah and colleagues[34] of histologic changes in gastrointestinal mucosal biopsies of 15 symptomatic patients with genetically confirmed SDS demonstrated that more than 50% showed varying degrees of duodenal inflammation by histology. This result suggests that there may be an enteropathic component in addition to the pancreatic exocrine failure contributing to the symptoms in some patients with SDS.

Although the pancreatic manifestations of SDS are well known, patients with SDS often have other gastrointestinal involvement, most notably in the liver. A recent longitudinal study of 12 Finnish patients with SDS further characterized the hepatic manifestations of SDS,[11] confirming previous reports of elevated levels of transaminases and hepatomegaly in younger patients with SDS that resolve with age. In addition, this study found that a majority (58%) of patients had elevated levels of bile acids. Of these patients, 3 had longitudinal bile acid measurements, and all had repeatedly elevated levels, although intermittently in 2, raising the concern for persistent cholestasis. Longitudinal examination of hepatic imaging revealed hepatomegaly only in young patients (younger than 3 years). Interestingly, all 3 patients older than 30 years had developed hepatic microcysts that were readily apparent on imaging studies.

SKELETAL MANIFESTATIONS

Skeletal dysplasias are also a frequent manifestation of SDS. The characteristic findings in SDS include short stature as well as delayed appearance of normally shaped epiphyses and progressive metaphyseal thickening/dysplasia in the long bones and costochondral junctions. In a group of 15 individuals with genetically confirmed SDS, Makitie and colleagues[9] demonstrated skeletal abnormalities in all individuals, although they were variable in severity and location, often evolving with age.

In a recent study, Toiviainen-Salo and colleagues[35] demonstrated that SDS is also associated with low-turnover osteoporosis. A total of 11 individuals with genetically confirmed SDS were evaluated and 10 were found to have abnormalities of bone health, including markedly reduced bone mineral density by Z-scores, with 3 individuals also demonstrating vertebral compression fractures. Mild vitamin D deficiency was present in 6 individuals, 3 with secondary hyperparathyroidism, while vitamin K deficiency was also found in 6 individuals, both of which are known to play an important role in skeletal health.

NEUROCOGNITIVE MANIFESTATIONS

Historically, patients with SDS have been shown to have neurocognitive impairment as well as structural brain alterations.[36,37] In a recent study, Kerr and colleagues[10] reported on the neuropsychological function in 34 children with SDS, comparing them to 13 sibling controls as well as 20 patients with cystic fibrosis matched for age and gender. Patients with SDS ranged widely in their abilities compared with controls, from severely impaired to superior in some areas measured. Overall, this study found that patients with SDS may have significant impairments in perceptual skills including reasoning and visual-motor skills, higher-order language, intellectual reasoning, and academic achievement. About 20% of patients with SDS were found to have an intellectual disability, with perceptual reasoning being particularly difficul. Furthermore, children with SDS were 10 times more likely to be diagnosed with pervasive developmental disorder (6%) than the general population (0.6%). In addition, both patients with SDS and their siblings were more likely to have attention deficits than patients with cystic fibrosis. These findings were not associated with secondary complications of SDS, sex, or age. It has therefore been postulated that SBDS may have a role in neurodevelopment, especially because many patients with SDS have abnormalities on neuroimaging. These findings also emphasize the importance of early neurocognitive assessment and intervention in patients with SDS.

DIAGNOSTIC APPROACH AND MANAGEMENT

Although the clinical diagnosis of SDS is often made in the first few years of life, typically with the classic presentation including failure to thrive, associated feeding difficulties, and variable recurrent or excessive infections, many patients may be diagnosed later in childhood or even adulthood, especially those with more mild pancreatic phenotype. It is important to recognize that older patients may present at a stage when pancreatic dysfunction is no longer evident, and thus a high index of suspicion may be warranted. The diagnostic workup continues to evolve, and the diagnosis is currently made clinically based on evidence of pancreatic dysfunction and hematologic abnormalities (see **Box 1**). Approximately 90% of patients with SDS have a biallelic mutation in the SBDS gene, leaving 10% without known molecular cause. It is important to consider other common causes of pancreatic dysfunction including cystic fibrosis, which can be ruled out with a sweat chloride test, as well as other inherited marrow failure disorders including Pearson disease, which includes pancreatic dysfunction, cytopenias, and bone marrow ring sideroblasts.

Patients with SDS require thorough screening for associated complications both at diagnosis and subsequently at regular intervals throughout their care. Recommended evaluations are listed in **Table 1**. Regular complete blood cell counts and bone marrow evaluations should be emphasized to monitor for the evolution of marrow dysfunction or malignant transformation, regular nutritional and growth assessments, as well as neurodevelopmental evaluations. Genetic counseling should be made available to patients as well as family members.

Surveillance as described above and supportive care for the complications of SDS are critical for the medical management of patients with SDS. Pancreatic enzyme supplementation should be administered to those with evidence of pancreatic insufficiency. Although many patients with SDS manifest varying degrees of cytopenias, regular transfusion requirements are rare outside the setting of severe aplastic

Table 1
Clinical evaluations for patients with Shwachman–Diamond syndrome

	Interval
Hematology	
CBC	Diagnosis, every 3–6 mo or as clinically indicated
Bone marrow aspirate and biopsy	Diagnosis, every 1–3 y or as clinically indicated
Fe, folate, B_{12} levels	Diagnosis, as clinically indicated
IgG, IgA, IgM levels	Diagnosis, as clinically indicated
HLA testing	As clinically indicated
Gastroenterology	
Pancreatic enzymes (trypsinogen, pancreatic isoamylase, 72-h fat excretion, elastase)	Diagnosis, as clinically indicated
Fat-soluble vitamins (A, D, E)	Diagnosis, 1 mo after initiation of pancreatic enzyme therapy; then every 6–12 mo
Prothrombin time (surrogate for vitamin K)	Diagnosis, 1 mo after initiation of pancreatic enzyme therapy; then every 6–12 mo
Liver panel	Diagnosis, as clinically indicated
Pancreatic imaging (ultrasonography)	Diagnosis
Growth/Skeletal	
Height, weight, head circumference	Yearly
Skeletal evaluation	Diagnosis, as clinically indicated
Densitometry	As clinically indicated, screen in adults
Neurodevelopmental	
Developmental/neuropsychological screening	Diagnosis and regular assessment at follow-up for school-aged children aged 6–8 y, 11–13 y, and 15–17 y

Abbreviation: CBC, complete blood cell count.

anemia. Although neutropenia is common, it is typically intermittent and often mild to moderate in severity, thus most patients do not require treatment with granulocyte colony stimulating factor (GCSF). Chronic therapy with GCSF should be contemplated in the case of recurrent invasive bacterial/fungal infections with concomitant severe neutropenia, with the goal of infection prevention. Individual patients may require only an intermittent schedule of GCSF or may need continuous daily treatment.

Hematopoietic stem cell transplantation (HSCT) should be considered for the treatment of severe aplastic anemia and is the treatment of choice for progression to MDS or AML in patients with SDS. Chemotherapy can be used as a bridge to HSCT in AML secondary to SDS; however, prolonged complete remission remains elusive with chemotherapy alone in SDS, and thus urgent use of HSCT is warranted. Historically, outcomes in MDS or AML in SDS after transplantation lag behind those of severe aplastic anemia, emphasizing the importance of regular surveillance with blood counts and bone marrow examinations.[38]

MOLECULAR PATHOPHYSIOLOGY

The SBDS protein has been associated with critical cellular pathways including ribosomal biogenesis,[39–42] microtubule stabilization,[2] and actin polymerization.[43,44] More recently, further murine studies suggest novel functions in stromal effects on the marrow microenvironment.[3,4]

SBDS AND RIBOSOMAL BIOGENESIS

Recent studies have further identified the structure of SBDS and provided additional insights into its interaction with RNA. The crystal structure of *Methanothermobacter* SBDS was elucidated to a 1.75 Å resolution by Ng and colleagues,[39] and the structure of human SBDS was determined by solution nuclear magnetic resonance. Supporting the interaction of SBDS in ribosome function, the localization of the SBDS protein to the nucleolus of human cells depends on active ribosomal RNA transcription, as evidenced by its diminution with low-dose actinomycin D, an RNA polymerase I inhibitor. SBDS-deficient lymphoblasts from patients with SDS are hypersensitive to actinomycin D, which can be abrogated with the addition of wild-type SBDS cDNA, supporting an underlying impairment of ribosome biogenesis. In keeping with yeast models, SBDS also associates with the large 60S ribosomal subunit, although a consistent defect in ribosomal RNA processing in fibroblasts of patients with SDS was not demonstrated.[40] SBDS was also demonstrated to associate with multiple ribosomal proteins in HEK293 cells including RPL3, RPL4, RPL6, RPL7, RPL7A, and RPL8, as well as nucleolin and nucleophosmin.[45] Mutations in *Tif6*, the yeast *eIF6* ortholog, rescue the slow growth phenotype of yeast deficient in the *SBDS* ortholog *Sdo1*.[46] In recent work by Finch and colleagues,[41] the crucial role of SBDS in ribosome biogenesis was further shown through its interaction with the GTPase elongation factor-like 1 (EFL1) in mice. This interaction results in the coupling of GTP hydrolysis by ELF1 to the release of EIF6 from the pre-60S ribosome subunit in an SBDS-dependent manner. eIF6 functions in 60S subunit biogenesis,[47,48] and its association with the nascent 60S subunit sterically prevents its association with the 40S subunit.[49,50] These data support a model whereby SBDS facilitates the joining of the 60S subunit to the 40S subunit for active translation through the formation of the active 80S ribosome.[41] The conservation of this function was later confirmed in *Dictyostelium* species.[42]

SBDS AND STROMAL MICROENVIRONMENT

Involvement of SBDS in both bone marrow hematopoietic and stromal cell functions has been demonstrated previously.[15] Recent work by Raaijmakers and colleagues[3] has revealed new insights into the role of SBDS in bone marrow stromal cells. Targeted deletion of *Dicer1,* an RNAIII endonuclease essential for microRNA biogenesis and RNA processing, in mouse osteoprogenitors resulted in reduced expression of *Sbds*, along with disrupted hematopoiesis with subsequent development of MDS and AML. Acquisition of several genetic abnormalities occurred despite intact *Dicer1*. Subsequent deletion of *Sbds* in mouse osteoprogenitors also induced bone marrow dysfunction with leukopenia, lymphopenia, and MDS, along with bony abnormalities, mimicking clinical disease.[3] In addition, microarray expression analysis of human SBDS knockdown cell lines by Nihrane and colleagues[4] reveal increased expression of osteoprotegerin and vascular endothelial growth factor-A, which are known to have effects on osteoclast differentiation, angiogenesis, and monocyte/macrophage migration. These data suggest that changes in the hematopoietic microenvironment due to decreased SBDS expression in stromal cells may play a role in promoting MDS and malignant transformation.

SBDS AND GENOMIC INSTABILITY

Evidence pointing toward an additional role for SBDS outside of ribosomal biogenesis and the stromal environment has also been demonstrated. Austin and colleagues[2] demonstrated that SBDS can be localized to the mitotic spindle of primary human bone marrow stromal cells. They were also able to show that lymphocytes and fibroblasts from patients with SDS have an increased number of multipolar spindles during cell division, generating increased genomic instability. Orelio and colleagues[43,44] demonstrated colocalization of SBDS with microtubules and the centromeres of the mitotic spindle, as well as the microtubule organizing center in interphase neutrophils. They were able to show decreased SBDS expression during neutrophil differentiation both in a human myeloid leukemia cell line and in primary human CD34+ cord blood progenitor cell cultures, as well as differential proliferation and differentiation of neutrophils in SDS cultures compared with that of controls.[43,44] Together, these studies suggest a role for SBDS in cell proliferation and cell division in the myeloid compartment, which may be reflected by the clinical phenotype of neutropenia and risk of malignant transformation in SDS.

OTHER MOLECULAR FUNCTIONS

Additional roles for SBDS have also been recently highlighted. Investigations by Ball and colleagues[45] suggest an involvement in DNA metabolism by demonstrating that FLAG (fludarabine, cytosine arabinoside, and granulocyte-colony stimulating factor)-tagged human SBDS copurifies with proteins implicated in DNA metabolism such as replication protein A1 (RPA1), DNA-dependent protein kinase (DNA-PK), histones, and X-ray repair cross-complementing protein 5 (XRCC5). Orelio and Kuijpers[43] also revealed a role for SBDS in actin-dependent cellular activities by showing that it colocalizes with F-actin and Rac2 in cellular protrusions of activated and adherent neutrophils from patients with SDS as well as a leukemic cell line. F-actin polymerization is also altered and polarization is delayed in these patient-derived neutrophils, perhaps indicating a role in actin-related processes, as reflected by their impaired chemotaxis.

SUMMARY

Many exciting advances in our understanding of SDS have occurred in the past few years; however, our understanding of the natural history and spectrum of disease, diagnosis, and therapy remain limited. Ongoing basic and clinical investigations on larger numbers of patients are crucial to better tie together our evolving comprehension of molecular function and clinical manifestations of this multiorgan disease to affect the treatment of patients with this rare disorder.

ACKNOWLEDGMENTS

The authors apologize for the omission of any references because of space limitations. The reader is referred to the reviews mentioned in the text for additional information. A.S. was supported in part by grants from the N.I.H., St. Baldrick's Foundation, and the Butterfly Guild.

REFERENCES

1. Goobie S, Popovic M, Morrison J, et al. Shwachman-Diamond syndrome with exocrine pancreatic dysfunction and bone marrow failure maps to the centromeric region of chromosome 7. Am J Hum Genet 2001;68(4):1048–54.

2. Austin KM, Gupta ML, Coats SA, et al. Mitotic spindle destabilization and genomic instability in Shwachman-Diamond syndrome. J Clin Invest 2008;118(4):1511–8.

3. Raaijmakers MH, Mukherjee S, Guo S, et al. Bone progenitor dysfunction induces myelodysplasia and secondary leukaemia. Nature 2010;464(7290):852–7. http://dx.doi.org/10.1038/nature08851.

4. Nihrane A, Sezgin G, Dsilva S, et al. Depletion of the Shwachman-Diamond syndrome gene product, SBDS, leads to growth inhibition and increased expression of OPG and VEGF-A. Blood Cells Mol Dis 2009;42(1):85–91.

5. Boocock GR, Morrison JA, Popovic M, et al. Mutations in SBDS are associated with Shwachman-Diamond syndrome. Nat Genet 2003;33(1):97–101.

6. Dror Y, Donadieu J, Koglmeier J, et al. Draft consensus guidelines for diagnosis and treatment of Shwachman-Diamond syndrome. Ann N Y Acad Sci 2011; 1242(1):40–55.

7. Burroughs L, Woolfrey A, Shimamura A. Shwachman-Diamond syndrome: a review of the clinical presentation, molecular pathogenesis, diagnosis, and treatment. Hematol Oncol Clin North Am 2009;23(2):233–48.

8. Huang JN, Shimamura A. Clinical spectrum and molecular pathophysiology of Shwachman-Diamond syndrome. Curr Opin Hematol 2011;18(1):30–5.

9. Makitie O, Ellis L, Durie PR, et al. Skeletal phenotype in patients with Shwachman-Diamond syndrome and mutations in SBDS. Clin Genet 2004;65(2):101–12.

10. Kerr EN, Ellis L, Dupuis A, et al. The behavioral phenotype of school-age children with shwachman diamond syndrome indicates neurocognitive dysfunction with loss of Shwachman-Bodian-Diamond syndrome gene function. J Pediatr 2010; 156(3):433–8.

11. Toiviainen-Salo S, Durie PR, Numminen K, et al. The natural history of Shwachman-Diamond syndrome-associated liver disease from childhood to adulthood. J Pediatr 2009;155(6):807–811.e2.

12. Donadieu J, Fenneteau O, Beaupain B, et al. Classification and risk factors of hematological complications in a French national cohort of 102 patients with Shwachman-Diamond syndrome. Haematologica 2012;97:1312–9.

13. Hashmi S, Allen C, Klaassen R, et al. Comparative analysis of Shwachman-Diamond syndrome to other inherited bone marrow failure syndromes and genotype-phenotype correlation. Clin Genet 2011;79:448–58.

14. Aggett P, Cavanagh N, Matthew D, et al. Shwachman's syndrome. A review of 21 cases. Arch Dis Child 1980;55(5):331–47.

15. Dror Y, Freedman MH. Shwachman-Diamond syndrome: an inherited preleukemic bone marrow failure disorder with aberrant hematopoietic progenitors and faulty marrow microenvironment. Blood 1999;94(9):3048–54.

16. Rosenberg PS, Alter BP, Bolyard AA, et al. The incidence of leukemia and mortality from sepsis in patients with severe congenital neutropenia receiving long-term G-CSF therapy. Blood 2006;107(12):4628–35.

17. Dale DC, Bolyard AA, Schwinzer BG, et al. The severe chronic neutropenia international registry: 10-year follow-up report. Support Cancer Ther 2006;3(4): 220–31.

18. Donadieu J, Leblanc T, Bader Meunier B, et al. Analysis of risk factors for myelodysplasias, leukemias and death from infection among patients with congenital neutropenia. Experience of the French Severe Chronic Neutropenia Study Group. Haematologica 2005;90(1):45–53.

19. Alter BP, Giri N, Savage SA, et al. Malignancies and survival patterns in the National Cancer Institute inherited bone marrow failure syndromes cohort study. Br J Haematol 2010;150(2):179–88.

20. Tamary H, Nishri D, Yacobovich J, et al. Frequency and natural history of inherited bone marrow failure syndromes: the Israeli Inherited Bone Marrow Failure Registry. Haematologica 2010;95(8):1300–7.

21. Vlachos A, Rosenberg PS, Atsidaftos E, et al. The incidence of neoplasia in Diamond-Blackfan anemia: a report from the Diamond-Blackfan Anemia Registry. Blood 2012;119:3815–9.

22. Singh SA, Vlachos A, Morgenstern NJ, et al. Breast cancer in a case of Shwachman Diamond syndrome. Pediatr Blood Cancer 2012;59:945–6.

23. Sack JE, Kuchnir L, Demierre MF. Dermatofibrosarcoma protuberans arising in the context of Shwachman-Diamond syndrome. Pediatr Dermatol 2011;28(5): 568–9.

24. Crescenzi B, La Starza R, Sambani C, et al. Totipotent stem cells bearing del(20q) maintain multipotential differentiation in Shwachman Diamond syndrome. Br J Haematol 2009;144(1):116–9.

25. Maserati E, Pressato B, Valli R, et al. The route to development of myelodysplastic syndrome/acute myeloid leukaemia in Shwachman-Diamond syndrome: the role of ageing, karyotype instability, and acquired chromosome anomalies. Br J Haematol 2009;145(2):190–7.

26. Cunningham J, Sales M, Pearce A, et al. Does isochromosome 7q mandate bone marrow transplant in children with Shwachman-Diamond syndrome? Br J Haematol 2002;119(4):1062–9.

27. Dror Y. Shwachman-Diamond syndrome. Pediatr Blood Cancer 2005;45(7): 892–901.

28. Dror Y, Ginzberg H, Dalal I, et al. Immune function in patients with Shwachman-Diamond syndrome. Br J Haematol 2001;114(3):712–7.

29. Aggett PJ, Harries JT, Harvey BA, et al. An inherited defect of neutrophil mobility in Shwachman syndrome. J Pediatr 1979;94(3):391–4.

30. Rothbaum RJ, Williams DA, Daugherty CC. Unusual surface distribution of concanavalin A reflects a cytoskeletal defect in neutrophils in Shwachman's syndrome. Lancet 1982;2(8302):800–1.

31. Hill R, Durie P, Gaskin K, et al. Steatorrhea and pancreatic insufficiency in Shwachman syndrome. Gastroenterology 1982;83(1 Pt 1):22–7.

32. Mack DR, Forstner GG, Wilschanski M, et al. Shwachman syndrome: exocrine pancreatic dysfunction and variable phenotypic expression. Gastroenterology 1996;111(6):1593–602.

33. Stormon MO, Ip WF, Ellis L, et al. Evidence of a generalized defect of acinar cell function in Shwachman-Diamond syndrome. J Pediatr Gastroenterol Nutr 2010; 51(1):8–13. http://dx.doi.org/10.1097/MPG.0b013e3181d67e78.

34. Shah N, Cambrook H, Koglmeier J, et al. Enteropathic histopathological features may be associated with Shwachman–Diamond syndrome. J Clin Pathol 2010; 63(7):592–4.

35. Toiviainen-Salo S, Mayranpaa MK, Durie PR, et al. Shwachman-Diamond syndrome is associated with low-turnover osteoporosis. Bone 2007;41(6):965–72.

36. Toiviainen-Salo S, Makitie O, Mannerkoski M, et al. Shwachman-Diamond syndrome is associated with structural brain alterations on MRI. Am J Med Genet A 2008;146(12):1558–64.

37. Kent A, Murphy G, Milla P. Psychological characteristics of children with Shwachman syndrome. Arch Dis Child 1990;65(12):1349–52.

38. Myers KC, Davies SM. Hematopoietic stem cell transplantation for bone marrow failure syndromes in children. Biol Blood Marrow Transplant 2009; 15(3):279–92.

39. Ng C, Waterman D, Koonin E, et al. Conformational flexibility and molecular interactions of an archaeal homologue of the Shwachman-Bodian-Diamond syndrome protein. BMC Struct Biol 2009;9:32.

40. Ganapathi KA, Austin KM, Lee CS, et al. The human Shwachman-Diamond syndrome protein, SBDS, associates with ribosomal RNA. Blood 2007;110(5): 1458–65.

41. Finch AJ, Hilcenko C, Basse N, et al. Uncoupling of GTP hydrolysis from eIF6 release on the ribosome causes Shwachman-Diamond syndrome. Genes Dev 2011;25(9):917–29.

42. Wong CC, Traynor D, Basse N, et al. Defective ribosome assembly in Shwachman-Diamond syndrome. Blood 2011;118:4305–12.

43. Orelio C, Kuijpers TW. Shwachman-Diamond syndrome neutrophils have altered chemoattractant-induced F-actin polymerization and polarization characteristics. Haematologica 2009;94(3):409–13.

44. Orelio C, Verkuijlen P, Geissler J, et al. SBDS expression and localization at the mitotic spindle in human myeloid progenitors. PLoS One 2009;4(9):e7084.

45. Ball HL, Zhang B, Riches JJ, et al. Shwachman-Bodian Diamond syndrome is a multi-functional protein implicated in cellular stress responses. Hum Mol Genet 2009;18(19):3684–95.

46. Menne TF, Goyenechea B, Sanchez-Puig N, et al. The Shwachman-Bodian-Diamond syndrome protein mediates translational activation of ribosomes in yeast. Nat Genet 2007;39(4):486–95.

47. Sanvito F, Piatti S, Villa A, et al. The β4 integrin interactor p27BBP/eIF6 is an essential nuclear matrix protein involved in 60S ribosomal subunit assembly. J Cell Biol 1999;144(5):823–38.

48. Basu U, Si K, Warner JR, et al. The Saccharomyces cerevisiae TIF6 gene encoding translation initiation factor 6 is required for 60s ribosomal subunit biogenesis. Mol Cell Biol 2001;21(5):1453–62.

49. Ceci M, Gaviraghi C, Gorrini C, et al. Release of eIF6 (p27BBP) from the 60S subunit allows 80S ribosome assembly. Nature 2003;426(6966):579–84. http://dx.doi.org/10.1038/nature02160.

50. Klinge S, Voigts-Hoffmann F, Leibundgut M, et al. Crystal structure of the eukaryotic 60s ribosomal subunit in complex with initiation factor 6. Science 2011; 334(6058):941–8.

Animal Models of Human Granulocyte Diseases

Alejandro A. Schäffer, PhD[a],*, Christoph Klein, MD, PhD[b]

KEYWORDS

- Chronic granulomatous disease • Leukocyte adhesion deficiency
- Severe congenital neutropenia • Neutrophils • Mouse models • Zebrafish models

KEY POINTS

- Human granulocyte diseases are mostly monogenic diseases affecting neutrophils, not eosinophils and basophils.
- Most monogenic neutrophil diseases are recessive or X-linked and can be classified as chronic granulomatous disease (CGD), leukocyte adhesion deficiency (LAD), or severe congenital neutropenia (SCN). Each of these can be caused by mutations in different genes.
- For CGD and LAD, mice bred to lack the orthologous gene mutated in each human form usually have a phenotype similar to that of the human patients. In contrast, for SCN, there is a striking discrepancy between the phenotypes of model mice and human patients.
- Not all animal models are mouse models. For some neutrophil diseases, there are naturally occurring models in dogs or cows. The construction of zebrafish models is an emerging trend in neutrophil diseases.
- Opportunities to characterize new monogenic forms of SCN, to generate new mouse models by random mutagenesis, to engineer new zebrafish models, and to use animal models in the exploration of new treatments should occupy researchers studying animal models of neutrophil diseases for many years to come.

INTRODUCTION

Granulocytes are immune cells that contain within them punctate granules, visible under the light microscope. There are 3 categories of granulocytes: basophils, neutrophils, and eosinophils, that are distinguished by whether they can be usefully stained by

Financial disclosure and conflicts of interest: None.

Funding: The research of A.A.S. is supported by the Intramural Research program of the NIH, NLM. The neutropenia research of C.K. is supported by grants from the Deutsche Forschungsgemeinschaft (DFG Gottfried-Wilhelm Leibniz Program), the European Research Council (ERC Advanced Grant), the Bundesministerium für Bildung und Forschung, and the Care-for-Rare Foundation.

[a] Computational Biology Branch, National Center for Biotechnology Information, National Institutes of Health, Department of Health and Human Services, 8600 Rockville Pike, Bethesda, MD 20894, USA; [b] Department of Pediatrics, Dr von Hauner Children's Hospital, Ludwig-Maximilians-University, Lindwurmstraße 4, D-80337 Munich, Germany
* Corresponding author.
E-mail address: schaffer@helix.nih.gov

basic (high pH), neutral (medium pH), or acidic (low pH) stains. Eosinophils may have several roles in host defense and have been most widely studied in asthma.[1] Both eosinophils and basophils have roles in promoting the Th2 responses needed to defend against parasitic infections.[1,2] However, a search of OMIM (Online Mendelian Inheritance in Man) shows no monogenic disorders primarily attributed to eosinophil or basophil dysfunction. By laboratory assays, humans have been found with a partial or total lack of peroxidase in eosinophil granules, but they have mild anemia or no phenotype at all.[3] Ohnmacht and colleagues[4] generated mice lacking basophils, which will enable targeted studies of human diseases in which basophils may be important. The immune function of neutrophils and their roles in disease are much better characterized than those of basophils and eosinophils, so neutrophils and their diseases are focused on entirely in this article.

Neutrophils are first responders at sites of infection and part of the innate immune system. Neutrophils can fight an infection by diverse weapons: phagocytosis of the infecting microbe,[5] poisoning the microbe with toxic peptides stored in the granules,[6] and wrapping the microbe in neutrophil extracellular traps.[7] More generally, neutrophils enhance inflammation and inflammatory signals that eventually call in macrophages, T cells, and B cells for a more long-lasting attack on the infection. Consistent with the paradigm that the innate immune system is more primitive than the adaptive immune system, all jawed vertebrates are thought to have neutrophils or neutrophil-like cells called heterophils, which can kill microbes by phagocytosis.[8,9] Even some invertebrates, such as flies, have neutrophil-like cells.[10] One reason eosinophils are thought be important for parasitic infections is that parasites, such as helminths, are too large to be killed by phagocytosis.[1]

Not only are neutrophils conserved across jawed vertebrates, but so are most of the known genes mutated in human neutrophil diseases. This evolutionary perspective suggests that it might be possible to model each human neutrophil disease of known monogenic cause by knocking out the corresponding gene in a mouse and characterizing the mouse phenotype. One could also hope to discover new human diseases by first studying abnormal mice that turn out to have a neutrophil disease. In a few cases, fish have been deliberately used instead of mice; also included are naturally occurring models of 2 diseases in dogs and 1 disease in cows.

Classification of Neutrophil Diseases

Most human monogenic neutrophil diseases can be classified according to the type of malfunction. Conditions in which neutrophil defense is inadequate because the number of circulating neutrophils are too low, as measured by the absolute neutrophil count (ANC), are called neutropenia. Chronic benign and ethnic neutropenias are not discussed, but the focus instead is on neutropenias that may start at birth and that are associated with severe bacterial infections, called severe congenital neutropenia (SCN). Diseases in which neutrophils fail to migrate properly to sites of infection are called leukocyte adhesion deficiency (LAD). Diseases in which neutrophils fail to carry out the oxidative burst function are called chronic granulomatous disease (CGD). Based on these layman's descriptions, one might imagine that SCN would be easiest to explain at a molecular level and CGD would be the hardest to explain at a molecular level; the causes of neutropenia would be most conserved across species and the causes of CGD least conserved across species. Surprisingly, the opposite is true for both measures of complexity. Therefore, relevant animal models are presented in the following order: CGD, then LAD, then SCN, from best understood to least understood. One rare disease, due a mutation in RAC2, is at the boundary of CGD and LAD and that disease is described in the LAD section. Two monogenic diseases that do not fit into this 3-part classification and some complex neutrophil diseases are described in a fourth section.

Over 20 years of animal case studies are summarized to address the basic evolutionary question: For which genes does conservation of the gene imply conservation of the phenotype when the gene is mutated? From the way the question is posed, one should expect that the phenotype is conserved for some genes, but not for other genes. Clinicians may wish to know when the phenotype is conserved because for those genes and only for those genes, animal models should be useful to understand the cellular mechanism of the disease and to test treatments.

CHRONIC GRANULOMATOUS DISEASE

CGDs are primary immunodeficiencies characterized by recurrent infections and inflammatory lesions called granulomas. The granulomas can occur on the skin or in the liver, lymphatic system, spleen, gastrointestinal tract, or genital tract. Mechanistically, CGD occurs because of a defect in the respiratory burst oxidase activity in neutrophils. More specifically, the nicotinamide adenine dinucleotide phosphate (NADPH) oxidase complex does not produce adequate amounts of superoxide and therefore killing of microbes is impaired.

There are 5 phenotypically comparable CGDs caused by defects in any of 5 proteins that participate in the NADPH oxidase complex. These proteins are traditionally denoted according to their approximate molecular weights: p22, p40, p47, p67, gp91; the "g" in gp91 indicates that this protein is glycosylated; often, a superscript "phox" is added to all 5 protein names, but the authors omit that. Defects in a sixth participating protein RAC2 lead to a phenotype that overlaps CGD, but because RAC2 has other functions, that phenotype is more severe and is better classified as a leukocyte adhesion deficiency. The gene names are shown in **Table 1**.

There are documented human patients with null mutations for 4 of the 5 types. For p40 deficiency, the only documented human patient has compound heterozygous mutations, one of which may not be null.[11] Most human CGD patients in North America and Europe are men with a mutation in *CYBB,* encoding gp91, because *CYBB* is on the X chromosome. The other forms of CGD are autosomal recessive and affect men and women equally.

Mice with definitely or likely functional null mutations exist for all 5 types. Knockout mice for p40, p47, and gp91 were deliberately engineered. Mice with a homozygous mutation in p67 were generated via a cross of known mouse strains.[12] Mice with a null substitution mutation in p22 were created by N-ethyl-N-nitrourea (ENU) mutagenesis.[13]

The reported phenotypes for gp91, p47, and p40 knockout mice generally correspond to the phenotypes of the most severe human patients, with 1 proviso. Mouse studies typically report on immune response to challenge by a small number of microbial

Table 1
Human genes mutated in chronic granulomatous disease and corresponding mouse models with a mutation of the orthologous gene

Protein	Gene	Human Mutation Reference	Mouse Model Reference
p22	CYBA	75	13
p40	NCF4	11	16
p47	NCF1	89	15
p67	NCF2	90	12
gp91	CYBB	91	14

species, whereas CGD patients must cope with a plethora of infectious prokaryotes. Granulocytes of gp91-deficient male mice produce no superoxide.[14] Clearance of infection by *Staphylococcus aureus* and *Aspergillus fumigatus* (2 infections commonly seen in CGD patients) was delayed in comparison to gp91-sufficient control mice. When gp91-deficient mice were injected with the irritant chemical thioglycollate, there was increased neutrophil recruitment near the site of injection.[14] p47-deficient mice produce no superoxide in neutrophils.[15] Despite the lack of superoxide, the knockout neutrophils have some capability to kill *S aureus* in vitro, but it is reduced compared with p47-sufficent neutrophils.[15] p47 knockout mice developed spontaneous infections and had significantly lower survival than heterozygous or wild-type mice.[15] Histologic post-mortem examination identified granulomas similar to those seen in CGD patients.[15] p40 knockout mice have a deficiency in production of reactive oxygen species in response to TNF-alpha and their neutrophils have difficulty killing *S aureus* in vitro.[16]

The mouse model for the p67 form of CGD was obtained and characterized as follows.[12] A back-cross of the C57BL/6J strain (used in many laboratories) to the wild MOLF/Ei strain leads to variability in susceptibility to salmonella infections. This variation is consistent with recessive inheritance of a single locus and can be mapped to a region of mouse chromosome 1 containing the *Ncf2* gene, encoding p67. Sequencing identified that the susceptible mice are homozygous for a R394W mutation derived from the MOLF/Ei strain. A human CGD patient with an analogous R395W mutation has been reported. A functional assay suggested that R394W leads to a deficiency in superoxide production, which is a hallmark of CGD.[12]

The most interesting of the CGD model mice is the one for p22 deficiency, which has a Y121H homozygous substitution in the protein.[13] These mutant mice have the expected immunodeficiency, which in this study was demonstrated by challenge with Burkholderia, another infection commonly seen in CGD patients. Surprisingly, the p22 mutant mice also have a balance disorder because of faulty gravity sensing in the inner ear, which has not been reported for human patients with the p22 form of CGD. The molecular explanation for the balance defect is that there are several oxidase-producing complexes that share the p22 subunit; these complexes use different homologs of the gp91 subunit to partner with p22. One of these complexes, called Nox3, is needed for the generation of otoconia, which are calcium carbonate crystals in the inner ear used for gravity sensing. In contrast to the balance problem, the mice have normal hearing. The Y121H substitution does not truncate the protein in principle, but in practice it leads to no (stable) protein being translated, although there is mRNA. Thus, it may be considered equivalent to a functional null for purposes of modeling.

LEUKOCYTE ADHESION DEFICIENCY

In this section, 3 diseases, often called "leukocyte adhesion deficiency," and a fourth one, which is called here "RAC2 disease," are discussed. The 3 LADs are usually distinguished by Roman numerals, I, II, III. There are mouse models for each of the 4 diseases, and additional nonmurine animal models for 2 of them. For RAC2 disease, there are 2 zebrafish models that may be more useful than the knockout mice.[17] There is one other nonmouse model for LAD type I, some Holstein cattle have a disease called bovine leukocyte adhesion deficiency (BLAD). The animal models for LAD are summarized in **Table 2**. LAD I, II, III have autosomal-recessive inheritance. RAC2 disease is in principle autosomal dominant because the observed human mutations are heterozygous, but the observed human mutation D57N occurred de novo in the affected children[18,19] and animal models suggest that biallelic null mutations of *RAC2* could lead to the same disease.

Table 2
Animal models for different types of leukocyte adhesion deficiency (LAD)

Disease	Human Gene	Model Organism	Mutation	Reference(s)
LAD I	*ITGB2* (CD18)	Mouse	Hypomorphic	21
LAD I	*ITGB2* (CD18)	Mouse	Null	22
LAD I	*ITGB2* (CD18)	Cows	D128G	23
LAD II	*SLC35C1*	Mice	Null	26
LAD III	*FERMT3* (kindlin)	Mice	Null and null only in chimeras and neutrophils	30,31
RAC2 disease	*RAC2* (D57N mutation)	Mice	Null	33,34
RAC2 disease	*RAC2* (D57N mutation)	Zebrafish	Morpholino or D57N	17

Leukocyte Adhesion Deficiency, Type I

The mildest, most common, and first described LAD is type I, due to biallelic mutations in the integrin gene *ITGB2,* which codes for the protein usually called CD18. The phenotype includes recurrent bacterial infections, periodontitis, delayed wound healing, and granulocytosis.[20] At the molecular level, neither the integrin β1 subunit nor its 3 α subunit partners come to the cell surface as they should, impairing neutrophil adhesion and chemotaxis. Two mouse models were generated[21,22] that reflect a range of human LAD I phenotypes, depending on the severity of the mutations in *ITGB2.* A first attempt to make a knockout mouse led inadvertently to a mouse with a low level of *Itgb2* expression.[21] The phenotype of the mouse with the hypomorphic mutation includes the following: mild granulocytosis, poor neutrophil mobilization to a chemically induced peritonitis model, and delayed rejection of heart transplants. The knockout mice have a more severe phenotype including leukocytosis, skin infections, alopecia, defective neutrophil adhesion and migration, and an impaired respiratory burst (resembling CGD).[22] Knockout mice inoculated with the bacterium *Streptococcus pneumoniae* have much more difficulty clearing the infection than wild-type controls and many of the mice die of infection.[22]

Cows with BLAD have a homozygous D128G substitution in ITGB2. The clinical symptoms overlap those of the human disease: high neutrophil counts, recurrent bacterial infections, periodontitis, and oral ulcers. Leukocytes of other types seem to try to compensate for a lack of innate defense by boosting levels of IgG. Chemotaxis and phagocytosis of affected granulocytes are severely impaired due to poor adhesion, whereas adhesion-independent functions are not impaired. BLAD is of economic importance in the dairy industry because some bulls used often in mating turned out to be carriers of the BLAD-causing mutation.[23]

Leukocyte Adhesion Deficiency, Type II

LAD II has a more severe phenotype than LAD I because it includes developmental delay and short stature.[24] LAD II is caused by biallelic mutations in *SLC35C1,* encoding a protein involved in the transport of fucose, one of the sugars involved in post-translational protein modification. This modification is surprising because there is no obvious connection between fucosylation and CD18 or other integrins. The use of fucose has been partly conserved and studied in a variety of eukaryotes and prokaryotes. Indeed, 1 of the 2 seminal human studies reasoned that fucosylation pathway genes are conserved between humans and worms and used a complementation strategy in *Caenorhabditis elegans* to find that biallelic mutations of *SLC35C1* cause LAD II.[25]

For LAD II, Hellbusch and colleagues[26] engineered mice that are homozygously null for *Slc35c1*, which encodes the ortholog of the protein mutated in human LAD II. Mice are born in 1/2/1 proportions, so there is no prenatal lethality. The knockout mice have leukocytosis, especially elevated neutrophils and eosinophils, and poor postnatal survival. The mouse weights are reduced. Leukocyte rolling flux fractions and velocity are significantly reduced, perfectly consistent with the human LAD II phenotype.

In addition to obtaining these phenotypic characterizations, Hellbusch and colleagues[26] used the *Slc35c1−/−* mice to gain insight into the pathways of fucose transport. *Aleuria aurantia lectin* (AAL) is specific for 3 types of fucosylation and can be used in vitro to show that Slc35c1−/− mouse embryonic fibroblasts (MEFs) have a defect in a fucosylation pathway. It was known from previous work that there are 2 pathways to obtain guanosine diphosphate-fucose for fucosylation: a de novo synthesis pathway and a salvage pathway. Fucose is needed in the endoplasmic reticulum (ER) and in the Golgi; the set of fucosyltransferases in those 2 organelles are nonoverlapping. Slc35c1 transports guanosine diphosphate-fucose only into the Golgi, not the ER. Nevertheless, the mouse phenotype can be improved (better weight and survival) by the administration of fucose, which must somehow get transported to the Golgi.[26] This statement suggests that there is an alternative mechanism of transport that is less efficient, but works better as the concentration of fucose increases. Administration of fucose to 1 human LAD II patient similarly improved the patient's condition, but for a different patient, the fucose treatment was ineffective.[24] Further mouse studies, perhaps using mice in which 2 fucose pathways are disrupted, could give insight into the function of Slc5cl and its dysfunction in LAD II.

Leukocyte Adhesion Deficiency, Type III

LAD III is a severe form of LAD that combines the immunodeficiency of LAD I with a severe bleeding disorder due to faulty platelet function. LAD III is caused by biallelic mutations in *FERMT3*, which encodes the protein kindlin 3.[27–29] The bleeding can be more problematic clinically than the immunodeficiency.[28] Analogously, *Fermt3* knockout mice die shortly after birth because of the platelet disorder, and the initial characterization of these mice does not consider granulocytes.[30] To address this limitation, Moser and colleagues[31] went on to generate *Fermt3−/−* fetal liver chimeras and neutrophils. Using these cells, they could show that the neutrophils have an adhesion deficiency.[31] They suggest that the granulocytosis in LAD III (and by inference in LAD I) seems to be a compensation for the inability of the granulocytes to adhere and migrate to infected sites.[31] They connected LAD III to LAD I at the molecular level by showing that kindlin 3 binds to integrin β$_2$, and they did integrin mutagenesis experiments to show that the NXXF motif at positions 764–767 is needed for kindlin-integrin binding.[31] Although LAD III is fatal if untreated, it can be cured with hematopoietic stem cell transplant (HSCT) in some cases[27,28] because *FERMT3*, unlike other kindlin-encoding genes, is expressed only in cells of the hematopoietic lineage.[29,30] One difference between the human LAD III phenotype and the knockout mouse phenotype is that human patient erythrocytes have a normal shape, but knockout mouse erythrocytes have an aberrant shape.[28]

RAC2 Disease

RAC2 disease is functionally related to LAD and has been reported in 2 human patients, both carrying de novo heterozygous D57N mutations.[18,19,32] The phenotype includes recurrent infections, abscesses, impaired wound healing, and lack of pus.

The protein is translated at half the normal level, but the D57N mutation has a dominant negative functional effect. In vitro, the patient neutrophils were deficient in polarization, chemotaxis, azurophilic (but not specific) granule release, and superoxide anion production.[18] The first patient was treated successfully with HSCT via donation from a sibling.[32] The HSCT process ablated the original bone marrow, so that posttransplant, the cells are 100% donor-derived. This stringency is important because D57N is a dominant-negative substitution.

RAC2 disease overlaps CGD phenotypically because of the role of RAC2 in the NADPH complex, explained earlier. The disease is more severe because RAC2 has roles in cell adhesion, cell migration, and other pathways.[33] Clarifying RAC2 functions and how they are disrupted in RAC2 disease is difficult because, in mammals, there are 3 paralogous members of the Rac subfamily of Rho GTPases that overlap in functionality and differ primarily by tissue expression.[33] Rac1 is ubiquitously expressed; Rac2 is expressed solely in cells of the hematopoietic lineage, and Rac3 is expressed mostly in the brain.[33]

Roberts and colleagues made *Rac2−/−* mice and Gu and colleagues[33,34] engineered various single-gene and double-gene knockout mice for the Rac genes. They showed that Rac2-deficient cells have a defect in adhesion to fibronectin.[33] The mice do not suffer from opportunistic infections, but are susceptible to *Pseudomonas aeruginosa* infection, if challenged.[34] *Rac2−/−* mice have leukocytosis mostly because of a threefold increase in the ANC.[34] Superoxide production is impaired in vitro, but in vivo it seems that Rac1 can substitute for Rac2 in stimulating superoxide production[34]; in the superoxide aspect of the phenotype, Rac2 deficiency matches CGD rather than LAD. Neutrophil chemotaxis is impaired and Rac2-deficient neutrophils had impaired spreading on surfaces after integrin ligation, which explains the similarity of Rac2 deficiency to LAD I.[34] Rac2-deficient cells also have a significant reduction in proliferation and a significant increase in apoptosis. Rac2-deficient cells have a defect in actin polymerization and they do not migrate in response to SDF1 signaling.

Recently, Deng and colleagues[17] developed zebrafish models for human RAC2 disease. First, they prepared a morpholino with impaired *Rac2* expression; second, they engineered a knock-in of the human D57N mutation. Both fish models show similar aberrant phenotypes, strengthening the evidence that D57N causes disease by a dominant-negative mechanism rather than haploinsufficiency. Either expression of Rac2D57N or the morpholino model causes a failure in wound healing because of impaired neutrophil chemotaxis. In both models, neutrophils fail to respond to a *P aeruginosa* infection. Both models show a defect in polarization, which can be visualized because of the transparent nature of the zebrafish. Both models show neutrophilia without increased neutrophil production, consistent with the human phenotype. Even more interesting, the Rac2D57N mutant was used to study a neutropenia syndrome, called warts, hypogammaglobulinemia, infections, and myelokathexis (WHIM) syndrome, as described in the next section.[35]

SEVERE CONGENITAL NEUTROPENIA

In SCN there is a primary immunodeficiency because the number of neutrophils in circulation is too low to fight infections adequately. In humans, an ANC less than 500/µl, when not infected or less than granulocyte colony stimulating factor (G-CSF) treatment, is considered neutropenic; some authors use a lower threshold of 200 when adding the adjective "severe."[36] Recombinant G-CSF boosts the ANC in most SCN patients[37] and some untreated SCN patients mount a partial response to infections leading to temporarily higher ANC. The receptor for G-CSF is encoded by the gene *CSF3R*, and as one might expect, knocking out the corresponding gene in mice leads to neutropenia (**Table 3**).[38] Therefore, it is surprising that no SCN patients have been reported with biallelic inactivating mutations of *CSF3R*. Instead, some somatic mutations have been reported in patients undergoing G-CSF treatment. That inactivating mutations of CSF3R should lead to neutropenia is supported by the surprising discovery of a family in which the phenotype of neutrophilia is associated with a heterozygous T617N mutation that leads to a constitutively active form of the receptor.[39]

Table 3
Mouse models mutating the orthologs of genes mutated or expected to be mutated in human SCN

Gene	Human Mutations/ Inheritance	Mouse Mutation	Reference for Mouse Model	Are Mice Neutropenic?
CSF3	None?	Null	92	Yes
CSF3R	Somatic mutations only(?)	Null	38	Yes
LYST	Biallelic/recessive	Null? (*beige*)	93	No?
LYST	Biallelic/recessive	Skip exon 25 (*gray*)	80	No?
ELA2	Heterozygous/ dominant	Null	94	No, but neutrophil function is aberrant
ELA2	Heterozygous mutations/ dominant	V72M heterozygous knock-in	95	No
ELA2	Heterozygous mutations/ dominant	G193X heterozygous or homozygous knock-in	76	No, but SCN can be induced by a proteasome inhibitor
AP3B1	Biallelic/recessive	Null (*pearl*)	96	No
AP3B1	Biallelic/recessive	Null (*bullet gray*)	81	No
RAB27A	Biallelic/recessive	Null (*ashen*)	97	Yes, after LCMV infection[44]
GFI1	Heterozygous/ dominant negative	Null	98,99	Yes
GFI1	Heterozygous/ dominant negative	N382S retrovirally induced in cultured cells	55	Granulopoiesis blocked, but no ANC measured because this model is in vitro only
SLC37A4	Biallelic/recessive	Null	100	Yes
SLC37A4	Biallelic/recessive	Null + cell transfer	101	Yes
G6PC3	Biallelic/recessive	Null	47	Yes
HAX1	Biallelic/recessive	Null	48	No
TAZ	X-linked	Knock down by RNAi	102	Some animals

For all rows, the symbol of the mouse orthologous gene is identical to the human symbol except that the letters after the first that are upper case for human become lower case for mouse (eg, human *HAX1* is orthologous to mouse *Hax1*). Unlike CGD and LAD, the mouse models for SCN are not necessarily neutropenic, so the phenotype correspondence in the rightmost column is noted. In several cases of syndromic phenotypes, the articles describing the mice make no mention of neutrophil counts. The genes are listed in the order of the first publication year for a mouse model related to each gene, with ties broken arbitrarily.

In the Introduction, the authors made the traditional distinction between defects of neutrophil function (CGD and LAD) and defects of neutrophil number (SCN), but this is an oversimplification. In some types of SCN (eg, Hermansky-Pudlak syndrome type 2 [HPS2]), those neutrophils that do circulate have a defective phagocytosis capability,[40] but this is not a necessary or sufficient condition for a diagnosis of SCN. Other qualitative defects of neutrophil granulocytes, such as reduced calcium flux,[41] may also be associated with SCN and contribute to the severity of the infections.

SCN Is Heterogeneous in Multiple Ways

Animal models for SCN known in 2006 were reviewed previously,[42] so the authors focus on more recent results in this article. Neutrophils are among the most primitive immune cells, but a surprising number of genes and pathways seem to interact to determine the ANC.[42,43] The heterogeneity manifests at several levels. At the level of inheritance, SCN can be dominant (eg, due to a mutation in ELANE, GFI1), recessive (eg, HAX1, G6PC3), or X-linked (eg, WAS, TAZ). At the level of phenotype, it had been traditional through approximately 2007 to distinguish between syndromic forms of SCN and nonsyndromic forms of SCN. Classical syndromic forms that have animal models include the following: Hermansky-Pudlak syndrome type 2 (HPS2) due to mutations in AP3B1, Griscelli syndrome type 2 (GS2) due to mutations in RAB27A, Chediak-Higashi syndrome (CHS) due to mutations in LYST, Cohen syndrome due to mutations in VPS13B, WHIM syndrome due to truncating mutations in CXCR4, and Barth syndrome due to mutations in TAZ (see **Table 3**; **Table 4**). However, as indicated in **Table 3**, the knockout mouse models for HPS2, GS2, and CHS are not known to have an inherent defect in neutrophil number or function. In all 3 cases, hypopigmentation is a more visible part of the phenotype and has received most of the attention. In the case of GS2, Schmid and colleagues[44] showed that Rab27a−/− mice are neutropenic when challenged with a viral infection; this is in line with the observation that GS2 patients may have intermittent neutropenia, especially coincident with viral infections.

The utility of the distinction between syndromic and nonsyndromic forms has been diminished since 2007 because it was discovered that, in humans, biallelic HAX1 mutations[45] or biallelic G6PC3 mutations[46] can cause either syndromic or nonsyndromic neutropenia. There are mouse models for both forms of SCN, but the relevance to the nonneutrophil symptoms differs. G6pc3−/− mice are neutropenic[47] but do not share the cardiac defects and urogenital defects and other dysmorphologies seen in some humans with G6PC3 deficiency. In contrast, Hax1-deficient mice[48] share the neurologic deficiencies of the HAX1-deficient patients,[45,49,50] but do not accurately model HAX1-deficient patients whose phenotype is limited to neutropenia.[50]

The Newest Animal Models for SCN

The recently characterized dog model for Cohen syndrome,[51] called "trapped neutrophil syndrome" (TNS) in the border collie breed, provides an example of the limitations of modeling complex human syndromes in inbred animals. Unfortunately for breeders

Table 4
Non-mouse models for SCN in which neutrophils were tested and shown to be deficient

Organism	Gene	Inheritance	Mutation	Reference
Dog (collie)	AP3B1	Recessive	Null	103
Zebrafish	CXCR4	Dominant	Transgenic expression of human mutation	35
Dog (border collie)	VPS13B	Recessive	Four nucleotide deletion; may not affect all transcripts	51

of border collies, the carrier frequency of the 4 base-pair deletion causing TNS is high (estimated at 0.04–0.08).[51] Fortunately for SCN epidemiology, this high carrier frequency makes it possible to identify many border collies that are homozygous for the TNS-causing mutation, but would not necessarily be brought to the attention of a veterinarian. Shearman and Wilton showed (their Table 3) that human Cohen syndrome patients[52] and border collies with biallelic mutations in *VPS13B* have variable phenotypes, despite the shared mutation and the highly inbred history of the dogs. Two differences are striking: (1) all the dogs have TNS, but not all human Cohen syndrome patients have SCN; (2) essentially all human patients have developmental delay, but fewer than half the dogs have developmental delay.[51,53,54]

The zebrafish model of WHIM syndrome[35] (see **Table 4**) is special because it enabled a proof of the unexpected result that the neutrophil aspects of RAC2 disease and WHIM syndrome are complementary. The "M" in WHIM stands for myelokathexis, meaning that the ANC is low because neutrophils are stuck in the bone marrow. In contrast, most other forms of SCN are due to excessive apoptosis of neutrophils that are not necessarily stuck in the marrow. Two diseases where granulopoiesis is defective are SCN due to *GFI1* heterozygous mutations[55,56] and the syndrome reticular dysgenesis, discussed in the next section. WHIM syndrome is caused by heterozygous, truncating mutations of the chemokine receptor *CXCR4*,[57] for which zebrafish have a homolog. Walters and colleagues[35] showed that transgenic expression of a human mutation in zebrafish embryos does lead to neutrophils being trapped. They went on to show that expressing the deleterious D57N RAC2 mutation has the surprising, beneficial effect of getting the neutrophils to move properly again. Thus, RAC2 disease and WHIM syndrome demonstrate an interaction between neutrophil-related proteins, which is an aspect of complex diseases that are covered in the next section.

Additional Discrepancies Between Human SCN and Mouse Models

Unlike CGD and LAD, there are discrepancies among the genes known to cause recessive neutropenia in human patients and knockout mice. In addition to the "No" entries in the rightmost column of **Table 3**, biallelic mutations in *RMRP*[58] and *C16orf57*[59] cause syndromic forms of recessive neutropenia in humans, but mouse models have not been documented. Mice with either *Bcl2a1*[60] or *Mcl1*[61] knocked out (the MCL1 model is a conditional knockout) have phenotypes that include neutropenia, but no humans having biallelic mutations in the orthologous *BCL2A1* or *MCL1* have been described. *Csf3* and *Csf3r* are listed in **Table 3** and have the same mouse versus human discrepancy. The prospect that new mouse models may facilitate the discovery of human SCN genes is a focus of the Discussion.

OTHER GRANULOCYTE DISEASES AND COMPLEX DISEASES

Two human monogenic diseases, CTSC deficiency and AK2 deficiency, which have animal models but do not fit easily into any of the 3 preceding sections, are discussed. This discussion leads naturally to some mention of complex diseases, where *CTSC* and p47 animal models have been characterized.

The first miscellaneous monogenic disease is called reticular dysgenesis or adenylate kinase 2 (AK2) deficiency. AK2 deficiency is the most severe variant of severe combined immunodeficiency disorder characterized by extreme paucity of T cells, B cells, and neutrophils.[62,63] Reticular dysgenesis is syndromic because it also includes deafness as part of the human phenotype. The immune part of the phenotype can be cured with HSCT shortly after birth.[62] Pannicke and colleagues[63] generated a zebrafish model in which the orthologous gene *ak2* was inactivated by a splice site morpholino, but the primary analysis of the fish was of lymphocytes, not granulocytes. The fish lymphocytes do not develop, as expected, from the human phenotype.[63] Although adenyl kinase activity is needed in most if not all cells, the phenotype of AK2 deficiency is specific to the immune system and the ear because, in these cells, the paralogous AK1 cannot substitute for the nonfunctional AK2.[63]

The second miscellaneous monogenic disease is a disease of aberrant neutrophil function. Papillon-Lefèvre syndrome (PLS) is caused by biallelic mutations in cathepsin C (current gene symbol *CTSC*, previously represented by the gene symbol *DPPI*).[64,65] The main symptoms of PLS are as follows: (1) severe periodontal disease and loss of teeth because of infections and (2) keratosis affecting hands, knees, and feet. CTSC is involved in activation of granulocyte serine proteases. The engineering of *Ctsc* knockout mice was described months before the publication of the first human mutations, but the study focused on nonimmune aspects of the mouse phenotype.[66] CTSC has a defined function in neutrophil killing of microbes and functional studies have shown roles for CTSC in decreased neutrophil chemotaxis, impaired neutrophil phagocytosis, and defective superoxide production.[64] Therefore, it is surprising that only some PLS patients are susceptible to infections.[64] Years later, it remains unclear whether the immune aspects of the PLS phenotype are associated with the specific mutation in *CTSC*, modifier genes, or nongenetic factors.

Although the *Ctsc* knockout mice were not directly helpful in characterizing PLS, they have been useful in studying complex inflammatory disease. Mice lacking *Ctsc* have a significantly lower risk of abdominal aortic aneurysms.[67] If *Ctsc*−/− mice are given wild-type neutrophils, the susceptibility is restored, showing that the aneurysms are due in part to the inflammation produced by neutrophil recruitment. The neutrophil inflammation leading to aneurysms is associated with increased expression of *Cxcl2*, whose expression is low in *Ctsc*−/− mice but becomes high when these mice are provided with wild-type neutrophils.

Mouse Models Pertinent to Complex Neutrophil Diseases

Two other studies of complex diseases and one of the genes/proteins mentioned previously concern p47 (a CGD protein from **Table 1**). Two mouse strains that have been studied for decades for the phenotypes of diabetes and obesity turn out to be homozygous for a mutation in p47 that eliminates superoxide production.[68] However, the mice were apparently not tested for immunodeficiency by microbial challenge. The variation in the diabetes and obesity phenotypes had been previously attributed to a mutation in the leptin receptor, which is on mouse chromosome 4. Interestingly, *Ncf1*, which encodes p47, is located on mouse chromosome 5, but it seems that the mutations cosegregate because of a combination of randomness and the structured nature of mouse breeding crosses. Whether the *Ncf1* mutation is relevant to the diabetes should be investigated by further crosses that unlink these 2 mutations on different chromosomes.

The mouse mutation of p47 was crossed into a different strain of mice susceptible to arthritis and leads to increased susceptibility to arthritis in that model.[69] This study also showed that the p47 mutation in the leptin receptor–deficient mouse leads to expression and translation of a truncated protein. The authors speculate that this abnormal protein may have some role in promoting autoimmune disease.[69]

DISCUSSION

Our review of animal models for granulocyte deficiencies gives a mixed picture. Most models for human monogenic granulocyte diseases are based on mice, usually engineered knockout mice. Sometimes the animal model phenotype mimics the human disease phenotype and sometimes not. In most cases, the discovery of the human gene has preceded a targeted attempt to create animal models. One notable exception is *G6pc3*−/− mice,[47] which were generated before the identification of any human G6PC3-deficient patients and highlighted *G6PC3* as a functional candidate located in the genetic linkage interval for the first multiplex pedigree characterized with G6PC3 deficiency.[46] In contrast, *Ctsc*−/− mice[66] were described a few months before the discovery that *CTSC* mutations cause human PLS,[64,65] but the mouse study makes no mention of any skin or tooth phenotype.[66] A recent study goes further to show that Ctsc−/− mice are not especially sensitive to Aspergillus infections.[70] Surprisingly, there are only 5 diseases covered in this review for which the characterization of the mouse model preceded the discovery of the first human mutation; the other 3 are the p40 form of CGD, LAD III, and RAC2 disease.

The contrast between the success with *G6pc3* and lack of success with *Ctsc* exemplifies the mixed picture. In the remainder of this Discussion, the approach of "first the good news" is taken by summarizing recent positive developments. Then, "the bad news" of gene-specific open problems is discussed, ending with some opportunities to use animal models for neutrophil diseases that to date have been largely missed opportunities. Perhaps, a clear delineation of open problems and open opportunities can steer future research toward the ultimate goal of making animals more relevant to the diagnosis and treatment of human patients with neutrophil diseases.

One of the more promising indications of progress in animal models is the recent development of zebrafish models, such as those for WHIM syndrome[35] and RAC2 disease.[17] Using zebrafish embryos, researchers can visualize the normal and aberrant functions of neutrophils directly.[71] The point that it is less expensive to house zebrafish, feed zebrafish, and mutate the genomes of zebrafish than it is for mice makes zebrafish models especially attractive. One opportunity that has been missed so far in this direction is the analysis of the neutrophils in a zebrafish model of Barth syndrome,[72] for which other nonimmune aspects of the phenotype were evaluated. In a few cases, such as Barth syndrome or LAD II, it may be possible to use invertebrate models, but this can be tricky because it is often the case that there is not a clear one-to-one orthology relationship among sets of homologous invertebrate and human genes.

The opportunity to study complex, polygenic diseases is perhaps the most positive recent development in the area of animal models for neutrophil diseases. In the previous section the interesting progress on *CTSC* and p47 in complex diseases was mentioned. However, a similar opportunity to study p67 in lupus and inflammatory bowel disease has been missed, so far. A recent study showed a strong association between the H389Q amino acid substitution and human lupus, especially childhood onset.[73] The H389Q variant leads to reduced superoxide production, although most lupus patients with this variant do not meet the diagnostic criteria for CGD. Another recent study showed that the R38Q amino acid substitution is associated with early-onset inflammatory bowel disease; this variant affects the interaction between p67 and RAC2.[74] The findings that mutations of 2 different members of the NADPH complex are associated with autoimmunity in mice[69] and humans[73,74] suggest further studies of the other members of the complex in autoimmune diseases. The distinction in the type of autoimmune disease is at least partly due to the p47 mouse mutation being backcrossed onto an arthritis-prone strain.[69]

Some Open Problems

The catalog of animal models for monogenic granulocyte diseases (see **Tables 1–4**) is extensive, but incomplete. Open problems about specific diseases include the following:

1. Are there any human patients with biallelic mutations in *RAC2*? If so, what is the phenotype?
2. Are there any human patients with the p40phox form of CGD and biallelic null mutations?
3. Why do human patients with the p22phox form of CGD not have problems with their balance?[13,75]
4. Why do many G6PC3-deficient humans have heart defects and urogenital defects, whereas G6pc3-deficient mice have nonsyndromic neutropenia?
5. Why do *pearl* mice and *ashen* mice have no defect in neutrophil number or function?
6. Why do *Elane* knockin mice have normal neutrophil counts, unless endoplasmic reticulum stress is chemically induced?[76]
7. If neutropenia-causing heterozygous human mutations in *GFI1* are knocked in to a live mouse, would the mouse be neutropenic as suggested by the cell culture experiments of Zarebski and colleagues[55]?
8. Is it possible to construct a model organism for HAX1 deficiency that has neutropenia, but no neurologic phenotype?
9. Is it possible to construct a knock-in mouse or fish model of the p67phox variants recently implicated in susceptibility to lupus or inflammatory bowel disease?[73,74]

What About ENU Mutagenesis as a Method to Construct New Animal Models?

In a generalization beyond single diseases, very few examples have been observed to illustrate 2 important opportunities of animal models of granulocyte diseases that are seen repeatedly for other diseases, including other immune diseases. These opportunities are the use of ENU mutagenesis to generate mutant mice and the use of animal models in pharmacologic experiments. Hundreds of mouse models for human monogenic diseases, including dozens of immune diseases, have been generated by ENU mutagenesis. The laboratories of Bruce Beutler (2011 Nobel Prize winner in Physiology or Medicine) and Chris Goodnow are renowned for ENU-generated mouse models of immune phenotypes.[77,78] Another massive ENU mutagenesis screen, including but not limited to immune phenotypes, was performed in the laboratory of Martin Hrabé de Angelis.[79] Therefore, it is disappointing to observe that the only ENU-derived models listed are for the p22phox form of CGD,[13] for CHS[80] and HPS2.[81] In the last 2 models (*gray* mice and *bullet gray* mice), the number and function of the mouse neutrophils have not been characterized.

A subtle advantage of ENU mutagenesis is that the mutated genes seem to be targeted at random. Therefore, there exists the possibility of characterizing a monogenic disease in a mouse before the analogous human disease is identified and without much prior understanding of the gene's normal function. However, this did not occur for p22phox, because humans with that form of CGD were described[75] before the mutant mice were generated.[13] Another advantage of ENU mutagenesis is that ENU mutates single nucleotides and, as a consequence, in many cases, the mutant gene can be translated to a full-length protein of aberrant function. These proteins with substitution mutations can lead to phenotypes that are milder, later onset, or even different from the phenotype of mice with the same gene/protein knocked out. Moreover, the specific substitution mutations observed in the ENU-generated mice can give insight into which parts of the protein are important for its function.

The prospects for ENU mutagenesis would seem to be bright for discovering new, monogenic forms of SCN because this disease has surprising locus heterogeneity[42] and can be defined by a well-established laboratory assay (ANC).[36] Progress in identifying new monogenic forms of SCN is slow, with only HAX1 deficiency,[45] G6PC3 deficiency,[46] and C16orf57 deficiency[59] found in the past 5 years. Among these 3 genes, only *HAX1* and *G6PC3* could explain some nonsyndromic cases, and most patients with nonsyndromic SCN sequenced for *HAX1* and *G6PC3* do not have mutations.[46,82,83] The approach of using human genome-wide association studies of variation of ANC has failed in the sense that loci near plausible candidate genes can be found to account for a small portion of the variation in ANC and those statistical associations can be replicated,[43] but, to date, the genes identified by genome-wide association studies have not been found to be mutated in human SCN patients.

Use of Animal Models to Test Potential Therapies

Because this review appears in a volume concerning clinical hematology, this article closes with this challenge: How can animal models of neutrophil diseases be used to develop new and better treatments for patients? SCN patients can be treated with G-CSF for the neutropenia, but the mortality rate from infections, leukemia, and other conditions remains high.[84] Among the diseases the authors covered, the current prospects for patients with LAD III and CHS are especially grim. As high-throughput drug screens and targeted gene therapy become increasingly used in general, one can hope that these technologies can be tested on animal models on the path to better treatments for human patients.

In the early years of this field, a mouse model for the p47 form of CGD was used to show the feasibility of somatic gene therapy.[85] This model and the gp91 model were used to investigate the mechanism by which interferon-gamma may be a useful treatment of CGD.[86,87] This question is important, because the use of interferon-gamma has been controversial, but the studies in mice came only after human clinical trials. Sadly, the authors could not find evidence that any of the monogenic animal models listed above has been used to test any drugs for that disease. The closest example is the relevance of *Ctsc−/−* mice to clinical trials of CTSC inhibitor drugs to inflammatory diseases.[88] Astute clinicians can be aware that if the dental, skin, or immune aspects of PLS start to appear, then CTSC is probably being inhibited more than is advisable.

The idea to use animal models to study the function of neutrophils or neutrophil-like cells is not new. Paul Ehrlich, co-winner of the Nobel Prize in Physiology or Medicine in 1908, discovered the stains that could distinguish neutrophils, basophils, and eosinophils under the light microscope. Ehrlich shared the prize with Ilya Mechnikov, who discovered phagocytosis in marine invertebrates. More than 100 years later, opportunities abound to use animal models in mice, zebrafish, and other species, to learn more about phagocytic neutrophils and their aberrations in human patients.

REFERENCES

1. Kita H. Eosinophils: multifaceted biological properties and roles in health and disease. Immunol Rev 2011;242:161–77.
2. Karasuyama H, Mukai K, Obata K, et al. Nonredundant roles of basophils in immunity. Annu Rev Immunol 2011;29:45–69.
3. Lepelley P, Zandecky M, Parquet S, et al. Total peroxidase deficiency in eosinophils: a report on twin sisters, one with a refractory anaemia. Eur J Haematol 1987;39:77–81.

4. Ohnmacht C, Schwartz C, Panzer M, et al. Basophils orchestrate chronic allergic dermatitis and protective immunity against helminths. Immunity 2010;33:364–74.
5. Dale DC, Boxer L, Liles WC. The phagocytes: neutrophils and monocytes. Blood 2008;112:935–45.
6. Segal AW. How neutrophils kill microbes. Annu Rev Immunol 2005;23:197–223.
7. Fuchs TA, Abed U, Goosmann C, et al. Novel cell death program leads to neutrophil extracellular traps. J Cell Biol 2007;176:231–41.
8. Styrt B. Species variation in neutrophil biochemistry and function. J Leukoc Biol 1989;46:63–74.
9. Lieschke GJ, Trede NS. Fish immunology. Curr Biol 2009;19:R678–82.
10. Qiu P, Pan PC, Govind S. A role for the Drosophila Toll/Cactus pathway in larval hematopoiesis. Development 1998;125:1909–20.
11. Matute JD, Arias AA, Wright NA, et al. A new genetic subgroup of chronic granulomatous disease with autosomal recessive mutations in p40^{phox} and selective deficits in neutrophil NADPH oxidase activity. Blood 2009;114:3309–15.
12. Sancho-Shimizu V, Malo D. Sequencing, expression, and functional analyses support the candidacy of Ncf2 in susceptibility to Salmonella typhimurium infection in wild-derived mice. J Immunol 2006;176:6954–61.
13. Nakano Y, Longo-Guess CM, Bergstrom DE, et al. Mutation of the Cyba gene encoding p22phox causes vestibular and immune defects in mice. J Clin Invest 2008;118:1176–85.
14. Pollock JD, Williams DA, Gifford MA, et al. Mouse model of X-linked chronic granulomatous disease, an inherited defect in phagocyte superoxide production. Nat Genet 1995;9:202–8.
15. Jackson SH, Gallin JI, Holland SM. The p47phox mouse knock-out model of chronic granulomatous disease. J Exp Med 1995;182:751–8.
16. Ellson CD, Davidson K, Ferguson GJ, et al. Neutrophils from p40phox-/- mice exhibit severe defects in NADPH oxidase regulation and oxidant-dependent bacterial killing. J Exp Med 2006;203:1927–37.
17. Deng Q, Yoo SK, Cavnar PJ, et al. Dual roles for Rac2 in neutrophil motility and active retention in zebrafish hematopoietic tissue. Dev Cell 2011;21:735–45.
18. Ambruso DR, Knall C, Abell AN, et al. Human neutrophil immunodeficiency syndrome is associated with an inhibitory Rac2 mutation. Proc Natl Acad Sci U S A 2000;97:4654–9.
19. Accetta D, Syverson G, Bonacci B, et al. Human phagocyte defect caused by a Rac2 mutation detected by means of neonatal screening for T-cell lymphopenia. J Allergy Clin Immunol 2011;127:535–538.e2.
20. Springer TA, Thompson WS, Miller LJ, et al. Inherited deficiency of the Mac-1, LFA-1, p150,95 glycoprotein family and its molecular basis. J Exp Med 1984;160:1901–18.
21. Wilson RW, Ballantyne CM, Smith CW, et al. Gene targeting yields a CD18-mutant mouse for study of inflammation. J Immunol 1993;151:1571–8.
22. Scharffetter-Kochanek K, Lu H, Norman K, et al. Spontaneous skin ulceration and defective T cell function in CD18 null mice. J Exp Med 1998;188:119–31.
23. Nagahata H. Bovine leukocyte adhesion deficiency (BLAD): a review. J Vet Med Sci 2004;66:1475–82.
24. Lübke T, Marquardt T, Etzioni A, et al. Complementation cloning identifies CDG-IIc, a new type of congenital disorders of glycosylation, as a GDP-fucose transporter deficiency. Nat Genet 2001;28:73–6.
25. Lühn K, Wild MK, Eckhardt M, et al. The gene defective in leukocyte adhesion deficiency II encodes a putative GDP-fucose transporter. Nat Genet 2001;28:69–72.

26. Hellbusch CC, Sperandio M, Frommhold D, et al. Golgi GDP-fucose transporter-deficient mice mimic congenital disorder of glycosylation IIc/leukocyte adhesion deficiency II. J Biol Chem 2007;282:10762–72.

27. Kuijpers TW, van de Vijver E, Weterman MA, et al. LAD-1/variant syndrome is caused by mutations in FERMT3. Blood 2009;113:4740–6.

28. Malinin NL, Zhang L, Choi J, et al. A point mutation in KINDLIN3 ablates activation of three integrin subfamilies in humans. Nat Med 2009;15:313–8.

29. Svensson L, Howarth K, McDowall A, et al. Leukocyte adhesion deficiency-III is caused by mutations in KINDLIN3 affecting integrin activation. Nat Med 2009; 15:306–12.

30. Moser M, Nieswandt B, Ussar S, et al. Kindlin-3 is essential for integrin activation and platelet aggregation. Nat Med 2008;14:325–30.

31. Moser M, Bauer M, Schmid S, et al. Kindlin-3 is required for β-2 integrin-mediated leukocyte adhesion to endothelial cells. Nat Med 2009;15:300–5.

32. Williams DA, Tao W, Yang F, et al. Dominant negative mutation of the hematopoietic-specific Rho GTPase, Rac2, is associated with a human phagocyte immunodeficiency. Blood 2000;96:1646–54.

33. Gu Y, Filippi MD, Cancelas JA, et al. Hematopoietic cell regulation by Rac1 and Rac2 guanosine triphosphatases. Science 2003;302:445–9.

34. Roberts AW, Kim C, Zhen L, et al. Deficiency of the hematopoietic cell-specific Rho family GTPase Rac2 is characterized by abnormalities in neutrophil function and host defense. Immunity 1999;10:183–96.

35. Walters KB, Green JM, Surfus JC, et al. Live imaging of neutrophil motility in a zebrafish model of WHIM syndrome. Blood 2010;116:2803–11.

36. Haddy TB, Rana SR, Castro O. Benign ethnic neutropenia: what is a normal absolute neutrophil count? J Lab Clin Med 1999;133:15–22.

37. Dale DC, Bonilla MA, Davis MW, et al. A randomized controlled phase III trial of recombinant human granulocyte colony-stimulating factor (filgrastim) for treatment of severe chronic neutropenia. Blood 1993;81:2496–502.

38. Liu F, Wu HY, Wesselschmidt R, et al. Impaired production and increased apoptosis of neutrophils in granulocyte colony-stimulating factor receptor–deficient mice. Immunity 1995;5:491–501.

39. Plo I, Zhang Y, Le Couédic JP, et al. An activating mutation in the CSF3R gene induces a hereditary chronic neutrophilia. J Exp Med 2009;206:1701–7.

40. Jung J, Bohn G, Allroth A, et al. Identification of a homozygous deletion in the AP3B1 gene causing Hermansky-Pudlak syndrome, type 2. Blood 2006;108: 362–9.

41. Elsner J, Roesler J, Emmendörffer A, et al. Abnormal regulation in the signal transduction in neutrophils from patients with severe congenital neutropenia: relation of impairs mobilization of cytosolic free calcium to altered chemotaxis, superoxide anion generation and F-actin content. Exp Hematol 1993;21:38–46.

42. Schäffer AA, Klein C. Genetic heterogeneity in severe congenital neutropenia: how many aberrant pathways can kill a neutrophil? Curr Opin Allergy Clin Immunol 2007;7:481–94.

43. Okada Y, Kamatani Y, Takahashi A, et al. Common variations in PSMD3-CSF3 and PLCB4 are associated with neutrophil count. Hum Mol Genet 2010;19:2079–85.

44. Schmid JP, Ho CH, Diana J, et al. A Griscelli syndrome type 2 murine model of hemophagocytic lymphohistiocytosis (HLH). Eur J Immunol 2008;38:3219–25.

45. Klein C, Grudzien M, Appaswamy G, et al. Deficiency of HAX1 causes autosomal recessive severe congenital neutropenia (Kostmann disease). Nat Genet 2007;39:86–92.

46. Boztug K, Appaswamy G, Ashikov A, et al. A syndrome with congenital neutropenia and mutations in G6PC3. N Engl J Med 2009;360:32–43.
47. Cheung YY, Kim SY, Yiu WH, et al. Impaired neutrophil activity and increased susceptibility to bacterial infection in mice lacking glucose-6-phosphatase-ß. J Clin Invest 2007;117:784–93.
48. Chao JR, Parganas E, Boyd K, et al. Hax1-mediated processing of HtrA2 by Parl allows survival of lymphocytes and neurons. Nature 2008;452:98–102.
49. Kostmann R. Infantile genetic agranulocytosis (Agranulocystosis infantilis hereditaria): a new recessive lethal disease in man. Acta Paediatr 1956;45(Suppl):1–78.
50. Germeshausen M, Grudzien M, Zeidler C, et al. Novel HAX1 mutations in patients with severe congenital neutropenia reveal isoform-dependent genotype-phenotype associations. Blood 2008;111:4954–7.
51. Shearman JR, Wilton AN. A canine model of Cohen syndrome: trapped neutrophil syndrome. BMC Genomics 2011;12:258.
52. Kolehmainen J, Black GC, Saarinen A, et al. Cohen syndrome is caused by mutations in a novel gene, COH1, encoding a transmembrane protein with a presumed role in vesicle-mediated sorting and intracellular protein transport. Am J Hum Genet 2003;72:1359–69.
53. Cohen MM Jr, Hall BD, Smith DW, et al. A new syndrome with hypotonia, obesity, mental deficiency, and facial, oral, ocular and limb anomalies. J Pediatr 1973; 83:280–4.
54. Norio R, Raitta C, Lindahl E. Further delineation of the Cohen syndrome; report on chorioretinal dystrophy, leukopenia and consanguinity. Clin Genet 1984;25: 1–14.
55. Zarebski A, Velu CS, Baktula AM, et al. Mutations in growth factor independent-1 associated with human neutropenia block murine granulopoiesis through colony stimulating factor-1. Immunity 2008;28:370–80.
56. Person RE, Li FQ, Duan Z, et al. Mutations in proto-oncogene GFI1 cause human neutropenia and target ELA2. Nat Genet 2003;34:308–12.
57. Hernandez PA, Gorlin RJ, Lukens JN, et al. Mutations in the chemokine receptor gene CXCR4 are associated with WHIM syndrome, a combined immunodeficiency disease. Nat Genet 2003;34:70–4.
58. Ridanpää M, van Eenennaam H, Pelin K, et al. Mutations in the RNA component of RNase MRP cause a pleiotropic human disease, cartilage-hair hypoplasia. Cell 2001;104:195–203.
59. Volpi L, Roversi G, Colombo EA, et al. Targeted next-generation sequencing appoints C16orf57 as Clericuzio-type poikiloderma with neutropenia gene. Am J Hum Genet 2010;86:72–6.
60. Hamasaki A, Sendo F, Nakayama K, et al. Accelerated neutrophil apoptosis in mice lacking A1-a, a subtype of the bcl-2-related A1 gene. J Exp Med 1998; 188:1985–92.
61. Dzhagalov I, St John A, He YW. The antiapoptotic protein Mcl-1 is essential for the survival of neutrophils but not macrophages. Blood 2007;109:1620–6.
62. Lagresle-Peyrou C, Six EM, Picard C, et al. Human adenylate kinase 2 deficiency causes a profound hematopoietic defect associated with sensorineural deafness. Nat Genet 2009;41:106–11.
63. Pannicke U, Honig M, Hess I, et al. Reticular dysgenesis (aleukocytosis) is caused by mutations in the gene encoding mitochondrial adenylate kinase 2. Nat Genet 2009;41:101–5.
64. Hart TC, Hart PS, Bowden DW, et al. Mutations of the cathepsin C gene are responsible for Papillon-Lefèvre syndrome. J Med Genet 1999;36:881–7.

65. Toomes C, James J, Wood AJ, et al. Loss-of-function mutations in the cathepsin C gene result in periodontal disease and palmoplantar keratosis. Nat Genet 1999; 23:421–4.

66. Pham CT, Ley TJ. Dipeptidyl peptidase I is required for the processing and activation of granzymes A and B in vivo. Proc Natl Acad Sci U S A 1999;96: 8627–32.

67. Pagano MB, Bartoli MA, Ennis TL, et al. Critical role of dipeptidyl peptidase I in neutrophil recruitment during the development of experimental abdominal aortic aneurysms. Proc Natl Acad Sci U S A 2007;104:2855–60.

68. Huang CK, Zhan L, Hannigan MO, et al. P47phox-deficient NADPH oxiase defect in neutrophils of diabetic mouse strains, C57BL/6J-m db/db and db/+. J Leukoc Biol 2000;67:210–5.

69. Hultqvist M, Oloffson P, Holmberg J, et al. Enhanced autoimmunity, arthritis, and encephalomyelitis in mice with a reduced oxidative burts due to a mutation in the Ncf1 gene. Proc Natl Acad Sci U S A 2004;101: 12646–51.

70. Vethanayagam RR, Almyroudis NG, Grimm MJ, et al. Role of NADPH oxidase versus neutrophil proteases in antimicrobial host defense. PLoS One 2011;6: e28149.

71. Colucci-Guyon E, Tinevez JY, Renshaw SA, et al. Strategies of professional phagocytes in vivo: unlike macrophages, neutrophils engulf only surface-assoicated microbes. J Cell Sci 2011;124:3053–9.

72. Khuchua Z, Ye Z, Batts L, et al. A zebrafish mdel of human Barth syndrome reveals the essential role of tafazzin in cardiac development and function. Circ Res 2006;99:201–8.

73. Jacob CO, Eisenstein M, Dinauer MC, et al. Lupus-associated causal mutation in neutrophil cytosolic factor 2 (NCF2) brings unique insights to the structure and function of NADPH oxidase. Proc Natl Acad Sci U S A 2012;109: E59–67.

74. Muise AM, Xu W, Guo CH, et al. NADPH oxidase complex and IBD candidate gene studies: identification of a rare variant in *NCF2* that results in reduced binding to RAC2. Gut 2012;61:1028–35.

75. Dinauer MC, Pierce EA, Bruns GA, et al. Human neutrophil cytochrome b light chain (p22-phox): gene structure, chromosomal location, and mutations in cytochrome-negative autosomal recessive chronic granulomatous disease. J Clin Invest 1990;86:1729–37.

76. Nanua S, Murakami M, Xia J, et al. Activation of the unfolded protein response is associated with impaired granulopoiesis in transgenic mice expressing mutant Elane. Blood 2011;117:3539–47.

77. Beutler B, Moresco EM. The forward genetic dissection of afferent innate immunity. Curr Top Microbiol Immunol 2008;321:3–26.

78. Cook MC, Vinuesa CG, Goodnow CC. ENU-mutagenesis: insight into immune function and pathology. Curr Opin Immunol 2006;18:627–33.

79. Soewarto D, Fella C, Teubner A, et al. The large-scale Munich ENU-mouse-mutagenesis screen. Mamm Genome 2000;11:507–10.

80. Runkel F, Büssow H, Seburn KL, et al. Grey, a novel mutation in the murine Lyst gene, causes the beige phenotype by skipping of exon 25. Mamm Genome 2006;17:203–10.

81. Blasius AL, Arnold CN, Georgel P, et al. Slc15a4, AP-3, and Hermansky-Pudlak syndrome proteins are required for Toll-like receptor signaling in plasmacytoid dendritic cells. Proc Natl Acad Sci U S A 2010;107:19973–8.

82. Xia J, Bolyard AA, Rodger E, et al. Prevalence of mutations in ELANE, GFI1, HAX1, SBDS, WAS, and G6PC3 in patients with severe congenital neutropenia. Br J Haematol 2009;147:535–42.
83. Smith BN, Evans C, Ali A, et al. Phenotypic heterogeneity and evidence of a founder effect associated with G6PC3 mutations in patients with severe congenital neutropenia. Br J Haematol 2012. http://dx.doi.org/10.1111/j.1365-2141.2012.09110.x.
84. Rosenberg PS, Alter BP, Bolyard AA, et al. The incidence of leukemia and mortality from sepsis in patients with severe congenital neutropenia receiving long-term G-CSF therapy. Blood 2006;107:4628–35.
85. Mardiney M III, Jackson SH, Spratt SK, et al. Enhanced host defense after gene transfer in the murine p47phox-deficient model of chronic granulomatous disease. Blood 1997;89:2268–75.
86. Jackson SH, Miller GF, Segal BH, et al. IFN-gamma is effective in reducing infections in the mouse model of chronic granulomatous disease (CGD). J Interferon Cytokine Res 2001;21:567–73.
87. Fernandez-Boyanapalli R, McPhillips KA, Frasch SC, et al. Impaired phagocytosis of apoptotic cells by macrophages in chronic granulomatous disease is reversed by IFN-γ in a nitric oxide-dependent manner. J Immunol 2010;185:4030–41.
88. Laine DI, Busch-Petersen J. Inhibitors of cathepsin C (dipeptidyl peptidase I). Expert Opin Ther Pat 2010;20:497–506.
89. Casimir CM, Bu-Ghanim HN, Rodaway AR, et al. Autosomal recessive chronic granulomatous disease caused by deletion at a dinucleotide repeat. Proc Natl Acad Sci U S A 1991;88:2753–7.
90. Nunoi H, Iwata M, Tatsuzawa S, et al. AG dinucleotide insertion in a patient with chronic granulomatous disease lacking cytosolic 67-kD protein. Blood 1995;86:329–33.
91. Dinauer MC, Orkin SH, Brown R, et al. The glycoprotein encoded by the X-linked chronic granulomatous disease locus is a component of the neutrophil cytochrome *b* complex. Nature 1987;327:717–20.
92. Lieschke GJ, Grail D, Hodgson G, et al. Mice lacking granulocyte colony-stimulating factor have chronic neutropenia, granulocyte and macrophage progenitor cell deficiency, and impaired neutrophil mobilization. Blood 1994;84:1737–46.
93. Nagle DL, Karim MA, Woolf EA, et al. Identification and mutation analysis of the complete gene for Chediak–Higashi syndrome. Nat Genet 1996;14:307–11.
94. Belaaouaj A, McCarthy R, Baumann M, et al. Mice lacking neutrophil elastase reveal impaired host defense against gram negative bacterial sepsis. Nat Med 1998;4:615–8.
95. Grenda DS, Johnson SE, Mayer JR, et al. Mice expressing a neutrophil elastase mutation derived from patients with severe congenital neutropenia have normal granulopoiesis. Blood 2002;100:3221–8.
96. Feng L, Seymour AB, Jiang S, et al. The β3A subunit gene (Ap3b1) of the AP-3 adaptor complex is altered in the mouse hypopigmentation mutant pearl, a model for Hermansky-Pudlak syndrome and night blindness. Hum Mol Genet 1999;8:323–30.
97. Wilson SM, Yip R, Swing DA, et al. A mutation in Rab27a causes the vesicle transport defects observed in ashen mice. Proc Natl Acad Sci U S A 2000;97:7933–8.
98. Karsunky H, Zen H, Schmidt T, et al. Inflammatory reactions and severe neutropenia in mice lacking the transcriptional repressor Gfi1. Nat Genet 2002;30:295–300.

99. Hock H, Hamblen MJ, Rooke HM, et al. Intrinsic requirement for zinc finger transcription factor Gfi-1 in neutrophil differentiation. Immunity 2003;18:109–20.

100. Chen LY, Shieh JJ, Lin B, et al. Impaired glucose homeostasis, neutrophil trafficking and function in mice lacking the glucose-6-phosphate transporter. Hum Mol Genet 2003;12:2547–58.

101. Kim SY, Nguyen AD, Gao JL, et al. Bone marrow-derived cells require a functional glucose 6-phosphate transporter for normal myeloid functions. J Biol Chem 2006;39:28794–801.

102. Soustek MS, Falk DJ, Mah CS, et al. Characterization of a transgenic short hairpin RNA-induced murine model of tafazzin deficiency. Hum Gene Ther 2011;22:865–71.

103. Benson KF, Li FQ, Person RE, et al. Mutations associated with neutropenia in dogs and humans disrupt intracellular transport of neutrophil elastase. Nat Genet 2003;35:90–6.

Index

Note: Page numbers of article titles are in **boldface** type.

A

Adenylate kinase 2 (AK2) deficiency, animal models of, 138–139
Animal models, failure of mouse genetic models to recapitulate neutropenia, 28
    of human granulocyte disease, **129–148**
        chronic granulomatous disease, 131–132
        discussion, 139–142
            ENU mutagenesis as method to construct new models, 141–142
            open problems, 141
            use to test potential therapies, 142
        leukocyte adhesion deficiency, 132–135
        other granulocyte diseases and complex diseases, 138–139
            CTSC deficiency, 139
            reticular dysgenesis (AK2 deficiency), 138–139
        severe congenital neutropenia, 135–138

B

Beta integrins, in leukocyte adhesion deficiencies, 101–104
Bone marrow failure, in Shwachman-Diamond syndrome, 118–120

C

C/EBPα transcription factor, lack of expression in congenital neutropenia patients, 76–77
Chronic granulomatous disease, **89–99**
    animal models of, 131–132
Clericuzio-type poikiloderma, with neutropenia, 51
Congenital neutropenia. *See also* Severe congenital neutropenia., epidemiology of, **1–17**
    classification by known gene, 4–6
    definition of, 2–3
    health indicators used in describing, 3
    organization of registries for, 7–10
        genetics, 8, 10
        incidence at birth, 8
        prevalence, 8, 9
    outcomes, 10–12
        malignant transformations and risk factors, 11–12
        morbidity with extrahematopoietic involvement, 11
        quality of life, 12
        risk of severe infection, 10–11
        survival, 12
CTSC deficiency, animal models of, 138–139

Hematol Oncol Clin N Am 27 (2013) 149–155
http://dx.doi.org/10.1016/S0889-8588(12)00239-0
0889-8588/13/$ – see front matter © 2013 Elsevier Inc. All rights reserved.

hemonc.theclinics.com

Printed and bound by CPI Group (UK) Ltd, Croydon, CR0 4YY

03/10/2024

01040442-0014